FURTHER PRAISE FOR *Patient Siggy*

"The chief use of illness is to remind us of the linchpins of life: the love of family, the blessings of community, the comfort of prayer, the beauty of place. Sigourney Cheek has used her reminder well, and responded with more than just a whisper of grace."

Christine Kreyling
Author, *Classical Nashville* and *The Plan of Nashville*

"I love Sigourney's spirit and her ability to communicate that spirit through words. In this memoir, she takes us to the waters of healing in a cyberspace odyssey. Then she lures us to go deeper into those waters through reflections as she sorts out life and death. Through it all she reminds us the water is good, and brings us to the essence of our creation. This book is a gift."

The Rev. Becca Stevens
Chaplain, St. Augustine's Chapel at Vanderbilt University
Founder, Magdalene House

"It happens with unbearable frequency: someone you know, someone you love has cancer. Most often, you react based on hesitation— not quite knowing how to respond, what to say, how to help. In *Patient Siggy: Hope and Healing in Cyberspace,* Sigourney Cheek, with outstretched arms, invites you into her heart wrenching, powerful, and direct encounter with cancer. Accept her invitation to learn to cope with serious illness. You will be uplifted by her story while discovering how to reach out when serious disease strikes someone close."

Beth Seigenthaler Courtney
Chairman/CEO, Seigenthaler Public Relations, Inc.

"Sigourney's openness and honesty in describing her journey with life-threatening cancer inspires all of us—friends, families, physicians, nurses, and patients. By the intentional use of journaling, cyberspace, hugs, and prayer, she strengthens her community to walk with her step-by-step."

Roy O. Elam, MD, Medical Director
Vanderbilt Center for Integrative Health,
Vanderbilt University Medical Center

Hope and Healing in Cyberspace

To Betty

Patient Siggy

with best wishes

Sigourney Cheek

Sigourney Cheek

Trade Paper Press

Patient Siggy: Hope and Healing in Cyberspace

For more information, visit www.patientsiggy.com.

Library of Congress Cataloging-in-Publication Data

Cheek, Sigourney
  Patient Siggy : hope and healing in cyberspace / Sigourney Cheek.
    p. cm.
  ISBN 978-1-59652-503-0

1. Cheek, Sigourney. 2. Cancer--Patients--Biography. I. Title.
  RC279.6.C54A3 2008
  362.196'9940092--dc22
  [B]
                              2008036491

Trade Paper Press
An imprint of Turner Publishing Company

200 4th Avenue North
Suite 950
Nashville, Tennessee 37219
(615) 255-2665
www.turnerpublishing.com

Cover design by Michael Penticost
Photographs on pages 15, 49, and 81 by Judy Nebhut are used by permission

Printed in the United States of America

09 10 11 12 — 5 4 3 2

To my husband, Jim, and to my family,
Jamie, Lisa, Jack, and Baker,
Daniel and Anne,
Matthew and Jessie,
and to my circle of friends in cyberspace
who surround me with their healing love.

Contents

Acknowledgments

I thank my dynamic doctors, John Greer, MD; Roy Elam, MD; John Sergent, MD; Bill Whetsell, MD; and the indispensable nurse practitioner, Ellen Tosh Benneyworth.

I thank Audrey Wolf, Beth Stein, Alice Randall, and Anne Taylor Doolittle, who encouraged me to keep writing.

I thank Kimberly Manz, Beth Seigenthaler Courtney, and Ginna Foster for setting up the launch pad.

I thank my friends Nicky Weaver, Connie Cigarran, Anne Whetsell, Linda Mason, Carole Hagan, and Barbara Schneider, who read and re-read my manuscript. I thank Connie Cigarran for organizing friends to sit with me during nine hours of chemo treatments, and Carole Sergent for organizing the meals waiting for me when I came home. They organized my life and gave me the gift of peace of mind. I thank my dear brother and sister-in-law, Kevin and Barbar Woods. I thank Dana Sherrard, Diane Hawes, Mary Jane Smith, Cindy Spengler, Anne Clay, Marcella Zimmerman, Caroline George, Janet Younts, Peggy Kinnard, Betsy Lewis, Sally Huston, Cindy Wilds, Em Crook, Sally McDougall, Becky Griffith, and Barbara Caldwell for their constant and nurturing support.

And I remember my oldest friend in Nashville, Susie Davis, who is still with us in spirit.

Blanket-of-Comfort

 acklend • aliceh • alicem • alicer • alynem • annm • anns • annw • annec • anneg • annek • annes • annemariem • annetd • annew • annellen • audreyw • barbarab • barbarac • barbaram • barbaras • barbaraw • beccas • beckyg • bellas • berties • betha • bethm • beths • betsyb • betsyl • betsyw • bettyb • bettyf • bettyjb • camillab • caroleh • carolen • caroles • carolineg • carolinegg • carolines • carolynt • caryr • catherineo • cathyb • cathyc • cathyj • charlies • charlottea • christineb • christinek • cindym • cindyr • cindys • cindyw • claired • colemanh • collinsh • conniec • conniew • craigf • cynthiac • danas • danielc • davidm • deand • debd • debbieg • delphiner • dennish • dianeh • donaldb • donnac • donnak • dorothyb • dorothye • dorryf • dotsiem • edieb • edieb • ediemeileenm • elaines • elizabethn • elizabeths • ellenb • ellenm • ellenr • emc • erink • farrellm • fayeh • florenceb • francesb • genem • geoffreyb • gingerp • giorgioc • gracieh • gunam • gusd • gwenb • hadenp • hannahl • harrietf • harrietp • hildam • hobbyh • hollyc • hollyw • honeya • hopes • irenew • jackb • jackieh • jamiec • janec • janew • janettes • janr • jans • janeb • janes • janety • jeannieh • jeffc • jennieg • jenniferj • jerryw • jillg • jimm • joans • joannec • joannek • joellew • johnh • johnr • joyceh • judyk • judyn • judys • judyw • julesb • juliaj • julial • julieb • julieg • juliew • katee • kateg • kathew • kathyf • kathyh • katieg • kayb • kayh • kays • kayee • kellyp • kendalli • kendricka • kimberlym • kristenw • larryl • laurac • laurar • laureny • leew • lesliew • libbyp • lindab • lindam • lindseya • lisac • lynnm • lynny • lynner • madgeb • magidb • micheleb • marcellaz • marcies • margieb • margiem • margob • margueritek • marief • markt • marleio • marlinp • mariannar • marshallc • marthap • maryanne • maryannh • maryannm • marybt • maryc • maryf • maryg • maryjanes • marys • marysuet • matthewc • melindaw • michaeld • mikek • missye • missyv • mistyh • mitasr • mortk • nancys • nancyw • nantsr • nazanint • nickyw • ninad • pamj • pamw • patriciad • patricias • paulac • peachesb • peggyc • peggyk • peggyp • peggyw • rachelb • rebekahw • reesm • rickh • roseg • ruthc • sallyh • sallym • sandrae • sandram • sandyb • scottit • stephaniei • suea • suej • susanh • susans • susieg • suzannev • tootyb • trishl • troym • varinab • vickyz

The Mission

A year of cancer and chemo is wrenching. Yet, from another angle, my struggle was exhilarating on every level.

Any cancer survivor can tell you a story about a life-altering experience. You stand at the door of death and then survive and have another shot at life. The rigors of treatment and joys of winning the war change who you are.

The day of discovery is etched into my brain. The sickening, suspended anxiety of the first doctor's visit sets the scene. The shock, the disbelief of the diagnosis, the horror of the cancer word, the grossness of the blood and needles and invasion of your body, and the knowledge that this is just the beginning leave you in a state of panic. The confusing medical terminology, the misery of knowing you are sick, the stark hospital waiting rooms full of people with jaundiced skin and no hair, the hours in antiseptic examination rooms, the interruption of your daily routine, and the resulting isolation become the focus of your day. Then family and friends rally to the call, offering comfort. People pray for you, and you try to find meaning behind the concept. If you open up to them you let in a powerful force, but you lack the stamina to respond.

Usually the zaps of chemo and slow recovery before the next round are a lonely experience. What prompted me to write my story is that I found a way of sharing my journey, of sharing the hard times and the heart tugs, the tears and the laughter. By happenstance, I found an antidote for the isolation of illness.

In the first week of discovery, I received three different diagnoses ranging from a benign "watchful-waiting" cancer to a five-to-eight-months-to-live cancer. In truth, I had the worst form of cancer with the symptoms of the mildest one.

So confusing. I was exhausted. I wanted my friends to be informed, but after one phone call about the latest doctor's visit, I'd have no energy for a repeat performance. My predisposition to share, to be open, was a godsend from the start. I created a contact list in my e-mail program and filled in the names of eighteen friends. I was nervous, almost scared, writing the first e-mail. In the South, we're supposed to be private about a personal crisis. We're supposed to shrug it off with, "I'm just fine," aren't we? (I've only lived here for thirty-eight years, so I'm a novice.) I thought hard before composing a short summary of my prognosis. Then, with the touch of a button, I sent the message out through my computer, and everyone on my list was instantly on the same page. I had exposed myself to my friends, and they loved having the curtains opened and being let in. They not only responded with enthusiasm, but also forwarded the message to other friends who e-mailed back and asked to be added to the list. By the next e-mail, the contact list was up to forty-five. My friends wanted to know when I was having a treatment, and then, how I was feeling. They wanted to keep in touch without invading my space and disturbing my afternoon naps.

Medicine controlled my cancer, but e-mail was my salvation, my lifeline to a close community of friends who shared my struggle. After my first short, hesitant message, I knew I was on to something. I knew the instant messaging, the twenty-four-hour access to the computer, and the informality of the dialogue created a world outside my bedroom where, still in my pajamas, I could keep in touch with an ever-growing network of friends. By giving away, I received in abundance.

I kept my messages upbeat. By presenting my struggle with a positive spin, my mind and body embraced the attitude as well. The messages my friends sent back were soothing, nurturing, and asking for more. As the list kept expanding, the writing back and forth evolved as well, delving deeper into the innermost secret parts of my life and their lives. Energy began to build. A community began to grow, a community of healing formed in cyberspace. The e-mail chain turned into a shared sacred circle. The positive feedback transformed into healing prayer.

By the end of the year, my contact group had evolved into 160 people. The list had started with close friends in Nashville, but soon expanded to include Christmas-card friends, friends of friends who were cancer survivors, friends from church, children of my friends, fellow volunteers and staff from various charities I support, acquaintances in cities across America, and friends in Europe.

Although a fairly recent phenomenon, communication through e-mails is a well-honed and commonplace tool in the workplace. School-age kids caught on quickly and now are fully engaged in their chat rooms. E-mail messaging is just hitting its stride among nonworking people in their fifties and sixties, the prime ages when illness begins to affect too many of our lives. Gilda's Club, a nonprofit organization supporting those with cancer and their families, offers a free blog site for cancer patients, but for me, the general access lacks the intimacy of a one-on-one e-mail chat.

My cyberspace community embraced me and kept me warm during a long, challenging year. It was therapy for me, but the greatest lesson I learned was the positive energy shared by everyone who was engaged in my recovery. It is my hope that this book will teach others about the power of communal prayer, of choosing a positive path to fight through serious illness, of sharing the struggle through writing, and the lifesaving power of community during crisis.

As I finish typing these lines, I hope my sacred community will expand further and even more people will benefit from the lessons learned. I maneuver my mouse arrow to the File icon and press Save just before the cat jumps up and starts walking across the keyboard. How appropriate, as my story begins with the cat.

The Cat

*T*he cat saved my life. The crisis and the cat clearly have a fluky connection. She started me on a course toward amazing, scary, and unimaginable events. The events seemed to be a coincidence at the time, but looking back, I'm not so sure. To think that an everyday encounter, a spontaneous cuddle, saved my life seems absurd, but over the last year I have learned to look at coincidence in a different way. Especially after Wynonna told me, "Coincidence is God's way of staying invisible." Now I know she's right.

But I'm getting ahead of myself. We need to start in early March, maybe late February, 2005. Before last February, I had never paid much attention to the date or timing of ailments.

It's a chilly winter morning. I'm not an early riser, but the phone rings before 8:00 AM. I hate that. I drag myself into the kitchen to fix coffee and bring a cup back to bed with the newspaper. While I am sitting with propped pillows, the cat jumps up to visit my chest. She purrs; I pat. Her paw touches my cheek; I scratch her head—our usual drill. When she jumps down, there appears to be a flea on my pillow. Closing my eyes, I brush it off. The cat has been outside during warmer days. The approaching spring means she needs to be sprayed.

The next day I count four bites around my neck, three on the left, one on the right. The day after that, two of them are swollen to the size of an egg. They all itch. I try not to scratch; I avoid mirrors.

The middle-age skin around my neck is not enhanced by additional lumps. I think about the flea.

A week later, the swelling has gone down, but the bites are still there and itch like crazy. A rummage through our remedy drawer produces creams with cortisone. The next week the bites are still there, and the lymph nodes under both arms have become sensitive. On the phone, my friend Mary Jane, who is always ripe with instant solutions,

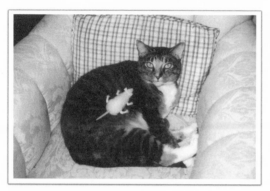

The cat, "Kitty."

suggests the lymph nodes are trying to fight off an allergic reaction. That makes sense, and then I try to think about something else.

The next week the bites change color: red rings with white insides. I scratch on either side of the lumps to avoid further irritation. Calling the doctor and asking for an antibiotic to end the misery occurs to me, but I have a busy week. I continue to pretend the bites are not there until Friday, April 7. That day I remember everything. The details and date are etched in my brain along with my wedding day and the birth of my first child.

I awake at 7:30 AM, roll over with my left arm wrapped around my pillow, and feel a significant pain under that arm. I get up, stand in front of the bathroom mirror, raise the arm over my head, and see a lump the size of an oblong grapefruit. What is going on? I calculate. I'm leaving for a week at the beach with my bridge group tomorrow. My husband, Jim, will come for the weekends on both ends. We return to Nashville for one night and are off again to New York for three days. That totals two weeks out of town. I circle the bedroom a few times, go back to the kitchen to start another pot of coffee, and go back to the mirror for a second look. That sucker is big. BIG.

I call our doctor, Roy.

"How are you?" he answered.

"You know I'm not terrific if I'm calling your office at eight-thirty in the morning on your cell phone."

I explain the bite, the lump, and the cat/flea theory. He asks if the cat scratched me. He mentions cat scratch fever as a possibility. "No scratches," I answer. He suggests I come in around eleven, there will be less of a wait. Roy was my parents' doctor. He is my father-in-law's doctor, my husband's doctor, our son's doctor, and has been a close friend for more than thirty years.

Roy's office is at the Vanderbilt University Medical Center: facility, huge; parking, daunting. I had not been to see Roy as a patient since his move to Vanderbilt more than a year ago. My body is so healthy that I rarely give it a thought. My parents didn't go to the doctor until they were in their seventies, and the strategy worked for them. As I ride around finishing morning errands, I realize I am overdue for an ob-gyn visit and mammogram, as well. I do try to keep some reasonable schedule for those two.

I pull into the Vanderbilt parking lot at 10:45 AM. I walk across the road to the main hospital entrance and step up to the information desk to learn that Roy's office is back across the road, above the garage. I should have called. I dodge traffic going back and make it to the seventh floor with five minutes to spare.

Four pages of clipboard forms go with me to the waiting room.

The perks of friendship have me in an examination room in fifteen minutes. Roy isn't as interested in my bites as he is in my lumps. He does mention that the bites could be lesions of some kind, not bites at all. "Do you mind if I bring someone else in to see you?"

"Ah, um, I guess not." My alarm system clicks on. Two other white coats come in to probe my pits. Then the three of them leave to discuss the situation behind my back as if I am out of the equation.

Roy comes back. He is concerned that both lymph nodes under my arms are enlarged. Did he say both? He thinks I should see a hematologist. What did that mean? Something to do with blood. He tells me the best person to see would be Dr. Greer, but sometimes it takes weeks to schedule an appointment. We discuss my scheduled departure in the morning. We talk about Florida. "I guess I could always fly back." I didn't want to cancel my trip, did I?

Roy leaves again and my mind goes to autopilot, hovering, until he returns. "I am going to walk you over to Dr. Greer's office. I'm on my way to lunch and the cafeteria is on the way."

We walk from Medical Center East across the second-story bridge to the hospital side. We walk through the back corridor of the hospital to the next building, the Vanderbilt Clinic. We talk about his son, Roe, and our doctor son, Daniel, and I try to focus on them instead of the doctor I am seeing in six minutes—who usually takes six weeks to see. We arrive at Suite 2603, the Hematology Clinic. Roy speaks to the scheduler about working me in, then hugs me good-bye and goes to lunch.

The lady at the desk adds more pages of forms to another clip-board, and I go to the waiting room across the hall. I can handle this. I ignore the people with baseball caps over bald heads as I fill out a record of fifty-nine healthy years, marred only by a hysterectomy in the early '90s. I ignore the person with the head scarf next to me as I quickly glance at, sign, and initial in several places the three insurance forms. I note the questions added since the last time I filled out forms: whether you feel safe at home, whether someone is threatening you. Because of my volunteer work at the YWCA Domestic

Violence Shelter, I am heartened to see these additions. The nurse later tells me they are directed toward the elderly. Unfortunately the caregiver usually accompanies the patient to the hospital, but occasionally the questions trigger a response.

I have brought William Manchester's *A World Lit Only by Fire* to read in Roy's office, and I take it out and turn to page 44.

Within fifteen minutes, the nurse calls my name. I go to another examination room and use my cell phone to call my husband, Jim. He had left at seven thirty this morning and didn't even know I was seeing Roy. Jim answers his phone on the second ring, and I tell him about the lump under my arm, the appointment with Roy, the move to a visit with a hematologist, and, yes, I'll call back the minute I have more information. Jim's law office is downtown and he could be at Vanderbilt in ten minutes, but I'm numb enough to be OK. I return to my book. Before I turn the page, Dr. Greer comes in. He is slender and sandy haired, in his fifties, with a soft, approachable smile. He checks my nodes. I tell him about the bites. He is noncommittal about any connection. He explains that he would like to take some blood samples. Depending on what they find, they might do a needle biopsy in one of the nodes as well.

I resist the impulse to turn around to see the person behind me to whom he must be speaking and concentrate on "needle biopsy." Maybe this is a movie. Maybe I am auditioning for a part. I fear I might be in the starring role. He sends me back to the waiting room until a technician comes to take blood samples. She takes me to a room the size of a small bathroom with shelves filled with plastic tubs, filled with plastic vials. No big deal, just a little blood drawn. Then she asks, "Do you have a port?"

The Diagnosis

The question moves me to center stage. I know what a port is. When my bridge friend Barbara was going through chemotherapy, she showed me this plastic thing they put under your skin so they don't have to insert a new IV each time you receive chemotherapy drugs. Why would I have a port? I take a breath and watch her count out vials. When she gets to fifteen, another alarm kicks in. The routine blood work with four vials is on another floor, in another building. She wraps the tourniquet too tight, then pricks the vein in my left hand and starts the vials. After about six, the blood stops flowing and she says, "the vein crashed." "My vein, what?" I want to ask out loud for clarification, but how can I talk with all those red tubes of my blood lying on the table? She pulls the needle out, picks up the tourniquet and wraps it tightly around my other arm, finds another juicy vein, and is off again for the remaining vials while I try to decide what is more painful—the tourniquet or the needle. I catch my breath and then ask how long she trained for her job. Two years and she has a six-year-old son. She smiles. Some of her salary went for gold fillings. I think of the women ready to leave the Domestic Violence Shelter and needing a job with a living wage. I remember the information that if you don't mind blood or failing bodies, hospitals offer a wide range of opportunities.

Back in the waiting room, a family of six is talking quietly about other people. They are a close-knit group that I sense have rarely been far from home. I imagine a farm three hours away. Where would they spend the night? A bald woman right next to me is having a conversation with a man who talks about the number of months he has left to live.

An elegant woman in a red pants suit comes through the door using a red umbrella as a cane. Right behind her, a young female doctor comes in and sits next to a forty-something patient. "You look fabulous," the doctor says. I glance sideways. The patient looks run over by a truck. What am I doing in here? Why am I sitting in the middle of this performance? I reread page 44 for the fourth time and contemplate out-of-body experiences.

A nurse calls me back into an examination room for a few more vials. On the way, I ask about where people stay who live too far away to go home. There is a hotel right across the street from Vanderbilt Medical Center with a sliding scale fee offering two-bedroom suites with kitchenettes for long-stay treatment. I feel better.

The nurse suggests that I grab a bite to eat in the cafeteria next door. I look at my watch as I cross the hall. It is two o'clock. I slide a tray down the row of options; nothing looks worth the effort to digest, but I assemble a small salad, pay the cashier, choose one of the few free metal tables, and nibble, trying not to think of my next meeting with Dr. Greer. Back in the waiting room, my name is called after a surprisingly short wait. Dr. Greer speaks in what is Greek to me about my blood. I get the part about pathologists coming in to do a needle biopsy. My immediate thought: If this invasion is necessary, wouldn't it be best to get it over with before the significance has time to kick in? I still want to look behind me when three white coats come in: the pathologist, an intern, and a medical student. The pathologist says he will take three needle samples. As he approaches me with a needle a foot long, he explains that over the years they have concluded that three is the magic number, not too few, not too many. He asks if I want the biopsy from the right or the left arm. I am shocked. Why wouldn't they automatically take the sample from the left arm with the larger lump? He explains that the cells are circulating through the lymph system and either side would show the same results. I don't get it and insist they invade the left side. Even though the spot is sore, why not go for the heart of the matter? The pathologist pokes three needles into my armpit, probing painfully around each time to collect misbehaving cells, while the pretty, blond intern holds my hand. I am so numb that the pain isn't that bad.

Then Dr. Greer tells me I can stay in the examination room until they have the results. I call Jim again. "Do you want me to come? I can be there in ten minutes." "I think I'm OK. Just come home as early as you can."

Why didn't I tell Jim to come, I wonder? My mind has found a protective zone where emotions are not invited. I am suspended in a safe place, like the waiting room. The consequences of all this testing are somewhere outside my reality. I just want to be home, in my garden. As I attempt the next page of my book, I imagine technicians in various labs sliding my blood and extracted node tissue under microscopes. At least we are not dealing with the challenges of the Middle Ages that William Manchester unveils. At least this is the twenty-first century. Besides, this is just a movie, and any minute the director will yell, "Cut!"

Dr. Greer comes back. My blood work looks good. He skims the sheet of indecipherable numbers and letters that might as well have been Egyptian hieroglyphics. He circles this and that. The good news—I am very healthy. Some of the cells in the biopsy look suspicious, however. They will need further testing: a CAT scan and a full-lymph biopsy.

Will that mean an operation? I have absorbed all I can handle. I'm not asking the question. "I guess we will be seeing a lot of each other," I say. Dr. Greer looks at the buttons on his white coat, and then his eyes move slowly up to my face. "You've had a long day." I look at my watch again and can't believe it is 5:15. I am grateful that I am already feeling good vibes about my doctor. I sense a gentleness, an empathy, a connection.

So much for thinking an antibiotic will clear up bug bites and return me to normalville. Dr. Greer says they will not have some of the results until later and he will call me at home. Jim will be on the phone with me to help interpret the next round, and that is a comforting thought. I thank Dr. Greer again for working me in, take my book, and drive home.

At the start of our street, I run into my daughter-in-law, Lisa, walking with her mother, Nancy, and the two most precious bundles on earth, grandson Jack, age two, and baby granddaughter Baker, age three months. A Jack fix is just what I need. His smile reaches into my heart. I pick him up, and rub his arm, as smooth as a flower petal, over my lips. I carry him to the jungle gym, behind the church on the corner. I put him down at the bottom of the slide ladder, and we all watch as his chubby legs carry him to the top. He laughs as he slides down and then runs around for another go, shouting, "See Jack." I give Lisa and Nancy a brief summary of my day and receive my first nurturing hug. Lisa is a slim, size 6 blonde with a gentle, loving touch. Those qualities come from her equally slim mom. Jim's and my joy is having our oldest son, Jamie, and his family a block away. We chat a while longer as I make a half-hearted attempt to explain my medical status, but fatigue soon has me back in my car for the ride to the end of the street and home.

At 5:45 PM I walk in the garden. The temperature is in the high sixties, and the afternoon light blankets the garden with a luminescent glow. The early, red peony leaves are unfolding like new butterflies. It is time to prepare bamboo cross stakes, a new system my gardener, another Jim, found a few years ago to hold the heavy blooms that will come. Copying is an art form that is encouraged rather than frowned on in gardening. I think of the seasonal rhythm of the exercise, the supply of bamboo that holds Christmas Amaryllis, winter *phalaenopsis* orchids, and then tall, spring and summer blooms. I have had some of the bamboo stakes for twenty years, and like old friends, they remain strong and reliable. I walk around the corner to the side porch off our bedroom. Two long strands of straw are on the chair under the edge of the arbor. I look up. The robin must have come back to the nest in the climbing roses that frame the porch. The baby robins will soon be chirping a welcome to spring, and the mama and papa robins will fly from the crepe myrtle tree to the wall that surrounds our garden and back with loud alarming calls each time we sit on the porch. They will fuss until the babies fly away. We will need to keep our voices low.

At 6:00 PM, Jim comes home. I wrap my arms around his lean, athletic body as he listens to another recap of my day. The warm, familiar smell of his shirt comforts me. I reach up to caress his strong shoulders. Even at sixty-three, his body is firm from a regimented two games of singles tennis per week, preferably at noon when the temperature is eighty and above. He loves to sweat. At 6:15, the phone rings. I introduce Jim on one end of the line to Dr. Greer on the other and another recap follows. "I usually don't give a diagnosis like this on the phone, but since we've been together most of the day I will go ahead, if that is all right with you." I murmur an OK.

"Your disease is a low-grade B-cell lymphoma." He talks again about some cells that are larger than usually seen with this diagnosis.

He talks again about my healthy blood. He says it would be OK to go to Florida tomorrow and says he will call back by Wednesday with additional information from the lab. I might have to fly back home. He gives me his pager and cell phone numbers, and says goodnight. How much should I read into acquiring Dr. Greer's cell phone number after one visit?

In one afternoon, I go from a healthy person with a clairvoyant cat and nasty bites to someone who is seriously ill. In less time than the robin spent preparing last year's nest for new eggs, my diagnosis has gone from a bug bite and an allergic reaction to a low-grade (whatever that meant) cancer.

You know what my first reaction is? "*Well, I better have more than an allergy after putting me through the ringer all day having tests.*" How dumb is that?

Where do I go to read about lymphomas? Medical terminology has never been my forte. The disbelief, the shock, the medical jargon I will have to learn are all hovering in my mind, and yet I still haven't really reacted. I am numb. I open a bottle of white pinot. The richness of my usual choice of red turns my stomach. I call Roy with an update and a thanks for getting me in to see Dr. Greer. I don't remember dinner, but I finish the bottle. I find an Ambien sleeping pill from our last overnight plane ride and gulp it down with the last sip, and sleep.

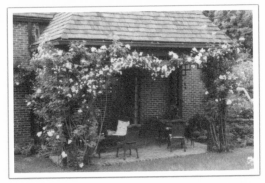

The side porch where I love to write.

The Grapevine

*T*he next morning, Friday, I still haven't cried. I still haven't told anyone else. I wake up remembering my mother falling off a ladder and breaking her leg in several places, followed by a hospital stay for two days, pins, and a big cast. She never said a word until she was home and recovering. I didn't feel protected—I felt pissed. What was family for? Vacations? I need to call my boys: Jamie, a block away; Daniel, in medical residency in Ohio; and Matthew, in the mountain town of Breckenridge, Colorado. Don't I?

My mind turns to Jim and his way of dealing with illness, and for the first time, it registers. I am not the only one with cancer. Jim was diagnosed with prostate cancer a year ago. For the first six months, only his doctors and I knew. While he consulted with three doctors in three cities, read everything ever written about prostate cancer, and contemplated possible avenues of action before deciding to go ahead with surgery in Nashville, he told no one, not even our three sons. I suspect that he consulted with doctor son, Daniel, but he doesn't pass on this information to me. Sometimes it drove me nuts, but I would remind myself it was his disease and his decision. I knew from thirty-eight shared years of marriage that Jim needed to come to any tough decision internally before sharing it with others. That is just the way his mind operates. That's one of the things that makes him such a good lawyer. I respected his right to deal with his illness his way, to say nothing of the fact that prostate cancer for any man is difficult to deal with, let alone acknowledge publicly. And now we both have cancer. Two extremely healthy people are both sick.

My mind switches back to the logistics of the day. Jim and I are leaving at noon for our place in Ponte Vedra, Florida, a grey, clapboard three-bedroom townhouse, spaciously designed with vaulted ceilings on the inside and weathered wood decks surrounding the outside. Built just behind the dunes that are constantly in flux from the pounding force of ocean waves, its views reach miles down the beach in both directions. Jim is staying for the weekend. My bridge group is coming for a yearly marathon from Monday until Friday, and then Jim is returning for another weekend. Not a bad buffer for bad news. Not a bad site to digest my diagnosis.

I think about sitting at the bridge table for five days with four women I have played with for thirty-six years. I am not Jim. Not mentioning the change in my life plan is highly unlikely. Once five ladies hear the news, the telephone lines will heat up. Bad news travels fast in Nashville. In my experience, it is not unkindly distributed. But a contest is in place, and there is some urgency to see who will be the first to know and who will be the messenger. People care about each other in our city. Many of us share a vast network of common friends and acquaintances. I feel tremendous support from the group. But before I leave, I want some control over the releases and I want to decide who will hear the news from me.

First I call Nicky, my oldest friend in Nashville. She and I are both Yankees who married into old Southern families, and we bonded thirty-eight years ago over the early challenges of assimilation. We even managed to have three children about the same ages, and they grew up as close as cousins, as close as siblings. On the phone, I cry for the first time. We talk a long time, and I give her the details of yesterday. She reminds me she had had similar tests several years ago, only to learn she had mono. Maybe my diagnosis was a false alarm.

Good try, Nicky, but I know my diagnosis is no false alarm. We talk about my departure and whom I should call before leaving. It would be nice to tell people in person, but my imminent departure has eliminated that option. The rest of the morning I call my closest friends and family. My oldest son, Jamie, called last night, soon after my encounter with his wife and children on the street, when I started gently with a few facts, a simple entry. This morning I start by leaving a message for middle son, Daniel, who is on call at a hospital in Columbus, Ohio. I leave another one for youngest son, Matthew, in Colorado. The bridge group could wait for Monday, in person. I call Carole, one of my oldest friends in Nashville, whose husband, John, is a doctor at Vanderbilt. Then she turns the phone over to John, "Will I have to do radiation?" "No," he says, "With this particular disease, you will have chemo." "Will I lose my hair?" "Yes." "I don't want to know that." "Then why did you ask me?" I call Connie, Mary Jane, Linda, Dana, all friends of thirty-plus years whose lives are densely interwoven with mine, layered with years of raising children, sharing trips and holidays, and informal Saturday night dinners. I call Anne, whose husband, Bill, is another doctor at Vanderbilt. I am collecting ammunition as well as spreading news. Connie, Anne, and I have an antiques business together called Amici. Our friends were skeptical about three, strong women going into business together, but we each bring different skills to the table. After eight years, our mutual respect and caring for each other has only grown deeper. The three of us share a powerful friendship.

Nicky comes over within fifteen minutes of my call. Her dark-brown hair is cropped short around a slender face with handsomely high cheekbones and a few too many age lines around her sparkling eyes from each of the years she has cared for a husband in a wheel-chair. Bill was diagnosed with MS (multiple sclerosis) more than thirty years ago. He fights his disease with a dignity and strength that has been both a privilege and a sorrow to observe. I know I will draw on that strength in the months to come. For the millionth time, I thank God for Nicky's friendship, our husbands' friendship, our grown children's friendships, and the start of our grandchildren's friendships. I have a flash of our two-year-old, Jack, and her four-year-old, Eads, jumping on the four-poster bed in her guest room, laughing and laughing, with Nicky on one side and me on the other standing guard to prevent a fall. Nicky and I try to find meaning in what is happening, but mostly we weep.

When she leaves the kitchen, the cat jumps on the table, rubbing her head on my hand, asking to be patted. The boys gave me the cat about six years ago for Christmas. She was a tiny tattersall kitten, and I named her Muff. I have a photo of her as a Christmas kitten, small enough to sit in the cluster of three blooming Amaryllis bulbs in the living room. Both the kitten and the plants had red bows. I thought the name appropriate until I noticed the boys looking sideways each time I said it. Apparently, an inside joke was floating over my head. Finally I confronted Matthew. He's always good for a straight answer. "Mom, that's a slang word for a woman's private part." Oops. The kitten had black rings around her eyes, so I renamed her Bandit. The name is on the vet records but somehow never stuck, and we call her "Kitty." No, not just "Kitty." Go up three octaves and say it again. That's it—a high "Keedy." Her ears prick up immediately; she meows and comes running. I make sure her water bowl is full, food ample, and litter tray clean before we leave the house for Florida.

The plane for Florida leaves at noon. Packing is a non-issue. A toothbrush, underwear, assorted pastel shorts, slacks, even the Revlon tinted moisturizer I find just as good as the more expensive Clarins are waiting in my closet in Ponte Vedra. With computer-printed boarding passes, we walk through the Nashville airport to the plane, board, land, and exit to the rental car without standing in any lines.

Perhaps the timing of this trip is another good coincidence. Our family has been going to Ponte Vedra just south of Jacksonville for over thirty years. Nicky and Bill's family have a house on the beach that we shared for two weeks each summer as the children grew. The first time, Jamie was about two. A photo of him in the water, naked, became a wedding rehearsal dinner show-and-tell favorite. In another picture, I'm very pregnant with Daniel. In a third, I'm not showing but remember being sick as a dog from the early stages of Matthew's conception. (Jim is a gifted picture taker.) In addition to visits with our friends, we have rented a variety of cottages on the Ponte Vedra beach, coming again at the end of the summer with assorted grandparents. About three years ago, we took the plunge and bought our own beach home.

On the plane, Jim and I talk strategies. He starts with a suggested medical plan: travel to other doctors in New York and do retests. He explains, "It's really important to have the tests redone at another hospital so the doctors there are interpreting their own findings, not someone else's." He thinks three doctors, three opinions are best. He reminds me of the importance of reading everything in print. I remember the two-inch-thick book on prostrate cancer on his desk at home. When he finally went in to discuss his operation with his doctor at Vanderbilt, he laughed about knowing more about prostate cancer and possible procedures than the doctors.

I say, "The thought of the same test in another city makes me choke." I read literature, not medical tomes. The conversation jumps two levels of intensity, and we are on the verge of an argument. Then we regroup. After thirty-eight years of living together, we end with a laugh about our differences, and realize we each need to make decisions in our own way about dealing with aging bodies and to respect our right to differ. I will turn my medical reading assignments over to Jim.

The plane lands in Jacksonville, and we take the pleasant route on Highway 9A, over the double-span bridge with silver poles rising hundreds of feet straight up, reflecting sun, spreading out like a sailfish to support the tons of suspended concrete decking as it crosses the St. Johns River.

In Ponte Vedra, we stop at the Fresh Market for our usual entry dinner of salmon on wilted spinach and drive the last leg to the house, five more minutes south. As we make our way up the weathered grey steps, the ocean salt and breeze surround my body. Inside, we open plantation shutters and doors to bring the ocean sounds inside while we put away groceries and listen to messages. Nothing is a chore down here. Jim and I may disagree about medical matters, but we are in agreement that the ocean is our drug to relax muscles and mind.

How blessed we are to retreat to the sea and let her magic work on any bad cells. Instead of sitting on the deck, I walk to the bedroom, flip back the spread, prop pillows, and burrow under the covers with my clothes on. Maybe I'm not my paternal grandmother who lived to be ninety; the time I have left floats by on the next wave. Regardless of the diagnosis, my life is in a different place from the last time I gazed at the sea. The bug bites itch, and I am constantly dabbing them with cortisone lotion and trying not to scratch. The soreness under my left arm is a constant reminder that my body is sending out alert signals. And I fear the pain will not fade away like the occasional neck aches from sleeping or sitting in the wrong position, the barely remembered monthly cramps, the swollen knees each spring from one mountain mogul too many.

I pick up *Time* magazine and read about the death of Pope John Paul II. Nancy Gibbs writes about the extraordinary vigil and endless line of waiting mourners. And then the author concludes, "Maybe it takes such a death for patience to be born." The article goes on to quote the Pope's last words to his private secretary, "I am happy. You be happy, too." How extraordinary to be able to say those words while dying, to know for certain that God will be waiting to greet you on the other side.

I need to stay in control, and to do this, I will need to make sure God is close by. I need prayer more than ever before, but what does prayer really mean? Should I pray for a spontaneous cure? And how would I feel if I didn't get one? Thoughts of prayer roll over me with each new wave. Instead of praying for someone else, my friends will be praying for me. I have already heard the offers. Viewed from the other side, being the recipient of prayer is a phenomenon I will have to digest one breath at a time.

In shorts, t-shirts, and bare feet, Jim and I sit on the deck before dinner, the cancer twins at the beach. We try to find meaning, put words to the strange disease that dwells in both of us. Was it the rose spray, the fake sugar, some mold under the house that we didn't even know was there?

We walk the beach each day at low tide. The only activities on the agenda are Jim's early morning outing for his newspapers, the *New York Times*, the *Wall Street Journal*, and the local *Jacksonville Gazette* (which will all soon form a large lump on the ottoman at the end of his comfortable chair), and his scheduled tennis game with the club pro at noon, when he can sweat.

The Bridge Brigade

On Monday Jim leaves and the bridge brigade descends in a ready-to-relax mode. The table in the front corner of the living room with serious ocean views is ready for serious cards.

The girls settle into the same rooms as last year. They hit the grocery on the way, and the fridge is stuffed with too many eggs, a mixture of milks, cereals, every variety of fruit, and four different brands of water so we can avoid using markers to identify whose is whose. I can't decide whether the latter is a good idea or the result of too many chiefs.

In short order, the bags are unpacked, travel clothes are discarded, and the cards are cut for the first round. I think about playing a few hands, but I need to lay the facts on the table before the cards. I am practically exploding with the untelling. The details of the day at Vanderbilt are told, and the retelling over the sound of surf spreads over me like a salve. Becky is a ten-year breast cancer survivor and the source of invaluable details. Susie's parents were both doctors, and she knows the lingo. Em says, "I knew something was wrong as soon as I saw your face," and uses her skills to find careful, comforting words. If I were home alone this week, instead of surrounded by a loving audience, I would drown with the absorption of the new data with no one to help analyze the lingo and options. For thirty-six years, these women have witnessed every birth, every loss of parent, every marital up-and-down, as well as an assortment of health issues.

As we dealt cards over decades, tallied scores, and triumphed over occasional slams, we honed our skills and friendships, and we are told, warded off Alzheimer's. Now it is my turn for center stage with no better audience to help me absorb and sort. I know that Jim could deal with any crisis internally or by going to a book on the subject for additional information. I need verbal venting, verbal feedback, the story to be told, tossed around, voiced from various perspectives. Maybe this is just a woman thing, but men are missing out. Each voicing heightens my awareness of where I am, and perhaps will help with how I proceed. Jim's processing is accomplished through reflection and reading, and he is impatient with my repetition of the same data over and over. I need my female team for continued verbal feedback.

Each day we deal cards after breakfast and walk the beach at low tide. At the bridge table, I am losing, low-man down. I am usually lucky at cards, but I decide my luck needs to be focused on those nasty lymphoma cells for the moment. On Wednesday, we take a break for a Beach Club Mayport Salad and shoe-store fix, but the rest of the time we dedicate to uninterrupted cards. At five-thirty each day, I hit the white wine, and for a few hours, the bad cells are forgotten.

On Wednesday night, Dr. Greer calls back. Becky knows the cancer vocabulary best and picks up the other phone with notepad in hand. I have already figured out that I need a second interpreter for these convoluted exchanges. Dr. Greer repeats much that had been said before the main message of the call is revealed: the diagnosis has changed. After more reviews of more tests and discussion with more white coats, the diagnosis is now CLL, chronic lymphocytic leukemia. He tries to explain the difference between leukemia and lymphoma, but I don't get it. A call back from son Daniel is perfectly timed, and he clarifies that white cells are born in the blood. Cancer cells in the blood are leukemia. Blood cells mature in the bone marrow. Bad cells in the marrow are lymphoma. So do I assume that bad cells in the marrow are more mature and more dangerous? Dr. Greer thinks the treatment might be "watchful waiting," but some of the lab work is still pending and he will call me back. He repeats the fact that there are larger cells than usually found with a diagnosis of CLL, but we are still possibly going to go with a "watchful waiting." No treatment, no hair loss. The best news is that Daniel has a free weekend and will fly down the next day, Thursday. In his second year of medical residency, he can act as in-house doctor for the first time. I also consult my extended medical team, Dr. John and Dr. Bill, my personal friends on the Vanderbilt campus in addition to Dr. Roy. They both report that CLL is better than B-cell lymphoma. I also give Bill and John permission to waive the HIPAA privacy violation, invade all my charts to their hearts' content, and chat with Dr. Greer. Due to the federal HIPAA privacy rule, they would not be able to do any of this unless I give permission. Interesting.

Daniel arrives Thursday night and is on the other phone for Dr. Greer's third diagnosis. The lymph biopsy results are back, and unfortunately, show a transformation to a larger, leukemia-type cell, with large sheets of B cells. The treatment has also switched gears. Dr. Greer explains they will do a chemo treatment, probably a mix of drugs including fludarabine, a wonder drug that has been extremely effective in fighting lymphoma and leukemia. "Would I lose my hair?" "Yes." I am, again, vaguely conscious of my underreaction to these changes in diagnosis. I ask Dr. Greer about the itchy bug bites and the pain going down my left arm, both annoying and constant. We also talk about my yearly mammogram being overdue. My files are at Baptist, another local hospital, but it now makes sense to have all cancer-related tests in the same place and all medical issues attended to in a timely manner, a strategy my formerly healthy body has always ignored.

I try to concentrate on the logistics of this unexpected plan instead of the consequences of hair loss, especially with the coming of summer, a special summer, a summer anticipated with excitement and fanfare—my sixtieth birthday celebration, a giant party week on the island of Mallorca, in Spain.

My mind turns to pleasanter thoughts. I grew up spending summers in Europe with my family. My father, an ancient art and archeology professor at Manhattanville College in New York, directed the excavation of a Roman colony on the island of Mallorca for forty-five years during the summers. While other children learned to paddle canoes and play tennis at camps and country clubs, I learned how Roman coins looked as they came out of the soil where they had been buried for two thousand years. I learned how the small, encrusted lump of dirt would miraculously transform after a night in a bath of acid, and Roman writing and the head of the reigning emperor would appear. As numerous coins were collected, the archeologists would have a historical record of the dates the city was occupied and by whom.

My soul was imbedded in the dry, dusty soil of the excavation, in the hot, summer sands of the coves around Pollença Bay. The bay keeps alive the name of the second-century-BC to third-century-AD Roman colony that had been named Pollentia. The bay where we would swim each day in the cool, turquoise waters for an hour before the two o'clock lunch at a long table that could seat up to twenty-four people in the Museum House in the nearby town of Alcúdia.

My father trained at the Institute of Fine Arts at New York University (NYU). He spent early apprentice years excavating in

Greece and then made a lucky connection with a wealthy philanthropist, William Bryant, from Vermont. Mr. Bryant loved all things Spanish and was fascinated by the expansion of the Roman Empire into the Iberian Peninsula, and the ingenuity and building skills that resulted in remains of their buildings still existing two thousand years into the future. During the Second World War, all archeological pursuits were put on hold. Many of the best archeologists were German and many were Jews. Luckily, they immigrated to the United States, and the center for archeological scholarship shifted to the Institute of Fine Arts at NYU where he studied. In the mid-'50s, Mr. Bryant was inspired to finance the start of a new excavation in Spain and offered my father the opportunity to be director. Daddy went to Spain knowing no Spanish, developed a network of Spanish archeologist colleagues, and learned of a potential site for an excavation in Mallorca.

There had been two Roman colonies on the island: a smaller one under the present capital of Palma, inaccessible to excavate, and a larger one on the other side of the island, under and around the small, sleepy town of Alcúdia. In the '50s, Daddy joined forces with two Spanish archeologists, pulled strings, and got permission to start a new excavation at the second site. The local people knew a city had been there. The Roman theatre was still nearby with huge, curved stone seats carved into the side of a hill. Over the years, farmers would occasionally dig up coins or pieces of pottery. Some of the largest marble statues had been rescued years ago and preserved in the museum in Palma. The village priest, Father Miguel, was Daddy's original contact. He had a pulse on the town, and people would come to him when they found an occasional coin or pottery shard or portion of walls. He was a frequent luncheon guest at our table, always in his long, black cassock, regardless of the summer heat.

The remains of a former civilization clearly lurked under the dirt that covered the fields on the outskirts of the small town. Alcúdia was surrounded by the remains of exterior walls and imposing arched entrance ways to the north and the south, all built during the Middle Ages. My father bought several fields just outside the walls of the town for the initial excavation. Only time and money and a team of experts were needed to unearth what remained of an even earlier civilization. Daddy acquired one of the largest houses in Alcúdia, put in plumbing and furniture, and renovated the second floor for archeologists and the third floor for students. We spent every summer in that small, walled city of about one square mile in size. My brother, Kevin, and I got to know the local kids. We learned where the post office, tobacco and stamp shops, butcher, and baker were located. None of the shops had signs. None of the streets had signs, except the name of the town as you entered, the *centro ciudad*, the center, which included a town square and the directions from the center to the next town. All the people in Alcúdia had lived there all their lives, as had their parents and grandparents. Nobody needed signs. The streets were a labyrinth and narrow, and the houses all looked similar on the outside. A hint of the prosperity behind the walls was reflected in the elegance or simplicity of the door knob and the wrought iron grate work on the upper floor windows. The seventeenth-century Museum House had an elegant pair of gooseneck brass knockers on an oak door wide enough to accommodate the horses and carriages that entered the interior courtyard fifty or so years ago.

When Jim and I married, my only assertive stance was to insist that "we will go to Mallorca every other summer." By the early '90s, both my parents had died. My only sibling, my brother Kevin, lives in

Madrid and has a summer house in Mallorca in a lush, green valley, sandwiched between two jagged mountain ranges behind the town of Pollença. After our kids were grown, I changed the Mallorca routine to every summer and the ten-day or two-week stay to one month. The month of August is now spent in Mallorca, as sacred a ritual as the real Christmas tree that touches our living room ceiling in Nashville for three weeks in December.

Over the years, dozens of our closest friends have visited and shared my beloved island and its magic, including Nicky, Susie, Connie, Dana, Mary Jane, and their families. Two years ago, six Nashville friends were together in Mallorca. They had such a wonderful experience that they started lobbying for a return visit. The house we now rent each August is on the edge of the Bay of Pollença, next to the beach where I have been swimming since I was thirteen. My friends and I sat at the long table on the terrace, watching the sailboats move in and out of the small marina to the right. Lunch was winding down. We were on Spanish time, about four-thirty, sipping the third glass of pre-siesta wine, when I had a flash. In two years, I would celebrate my sixtieth birthday, and I had been thinking of a big party in Nashville. But what if I invited my nearest and dearest to come to Mallorca for a week instead? Like many of our children's weddings, I could create a destination cele-bration. The idea was born over that lunch, and now, two years later, preparations had been made for the arrival of thirty-four friends to gather in three nearby small hotels for a much-talked-about and anticipated event in August 2005.

As I hang up the phone in Florida, I picture myself dripping from a pre-lunch plunge in the sea with hair slicked back and left to air dry at the lunch table, my version of Mallorca air-conditioning. I picture myself diving off my brother's antique fishing boat into the cool, crisp water before a picnic lunch topside. I think of all the picture ops during the up and coming celebration week. I imagine the swims with a rubber bathing cap, with a scarf, with a wig? How can I reign at my big birthday celebration with NO HAIR?

Back in Ponte Vedra, we sit down at the bridge table, but the card shuffling stops as we try to make sense of the latest "diagnosis of the day." The worst is a follow-up call from the scheduler at the hospital for a bone-marrow biopsy, a CAT scan, the full-lymph biopsy, and an MRI. Setting an exact date for the medical invasions makes my brain churn. My heart pounds as if it were slapped by the wet sand, battered by waves beyond the terrace. I will be going back for more tests on more machines. Looking down at the list of procedures I have just recorded moves reality too close and sets off flowing tears. So much for never going to the doctor; I am making up triple time. Dr. Roy calls in a prescription for more Ambien. Golly, I get fifteen pills instead of the travel pack of two. I can't compute the added attention to infirmities, but I can pour more wine. When anxiety or fear try to take over, I talk to a friend, fill a wine glass, or take a pill. Plan A: be pickled and avoid pain.

Jim comes back midday Friday, and even though we have gone over it before on the phone, I fill him in on diagnosis three. He sits down at his desk in our bedroom, opens the Internet on the computer, searches, reads, prints, mumbles, and then dumps stuff in the wastebasket. "What's that?" I ask. "Don't read it, it's not about you." Yeah, dangle a carrot and I won't become the donkey? When he leaves the room, I walk over and fish through the trash. I shouldn't have. A transformation from leukemia to a larger-cell lymphoma is called Richter's syndrome. Prognosis: five to eight months.

Holy shit.

I crawl into bed, curl up tight, pretend to be the cat with my head hidden in fur. My insides are tumbling, caught in the undertow. I think back. Dr. Greer has said I was atypical. I have none of the usual symptoms of people with this disease. The printout says people with Richter's syndrome are seriously ill before diagnosis. People with Richter's syndrome have had CLL for a long time, infected lymph nodes in various parts of the body, and blood counts off the charts. My blood work is practically normal. I am healthy. I can purr. I can't have that bad disease. But the "D" word has now been added to my radar screen, right next to the "C" word.

Dr. Roy calls. Jim asks if the "sheets of larger B cells" mean I have Richter's syndrome. Roy confirms the diagnosis. The assured longevity my parents enjoyed is sinking. The rest of my life has just shifted with the outgoing tide.

Jim and Daniel and I spend the rest of the weekend quietly walking the beach, eating seafood, trying to make some sense out of complicated cancer issues. Even with Daniel's medical degree to help, so much is left unsettled, unresolved, suspended.

Next Stop, New York

$\mathscr{O}$n Sunday evening, we return to Nashville, repack bags, and on Monday, we leave for a long-planned business trip of Jim's in New York. On the plane, Jim and I laugh about the words people have been using to describe my "situation," my "medical condition," my "medical challenges," my "medical issues." Cancer and death are interpreted with other words, and the other words are spoken in hushed tones. As a patient, I want to confront the word cancer. Something about saying it out loud removes the mystery. I make a mental note to use the word, hoping it will lose its sting. Why do we pretend cancer doesn't exist, the way sex and certain body parts didn't exist for our parents and our grandparents?

On Tuesday, I meet another old friend, Diane, for lunch at a small restaurant on Seventy-second Street. In the '70s, when I was in the hospital recovering from Daniel's birth, Jim went to a Vanderbilt Law School reception for new faculty members. He was on the faculty of the law school for the first four years of our marriage and before going into private practice with one of the largest firms in Nashville. After the reception, he came to the hospital and said, "You are going to love two of the wives of new faculty members." One was Dana, my friend who was in Mallorca two years ago, and the other was Diane; both are still two of my closest friends. Diane has always had a powerful faith. She is one of the few friends I can speak candidly with about all things spiritual. Do I tell her? Do I spend a few hours over lunch with a close friend and not tell her, wait for her to hear it from someone else? Diane is a Christian Scientist. In Christian Science faith, illness is an illusion. I decide to save my diagnosis for dessert. She digests cut fruit and information, taking her time to respond. We plan to tour the newly renovated MOMA, the Museum of Modern Art. She says, "Let's take the bus." I haven't been on a bus in New York since I lived here in my twenties. "A bus?" "Come on, New Yorkers are tired of the ever-increasing taxi fares. This is our way to protest." She pulls my arm, and within five minutes, we are bumping along. Heading downtown on Fifth, we sit high up enough to see people walking around the zoo in Central Park. I remember Saturday visits to the zoo with Jim when we both lived in the city. He was a summer clerk at Sherman and Sterling in New York when we first met at a party, and I was the native New Yorker. Now Jim spends far more time up here than I do. I couldn't remember the last time I had been to the wonderful, little Central Park Zoo. I tell myself that someday soon I will bring grandson Jack.

Diane and I avoid the subject of disease as she tells me a story. Years ago, in a snowstorm, Dustin Hoffman and Robert Redford were trying to catch a cab on the Upper East Side. With snow falling at a blinding speed, their attempts were in vain. Finally Dustin said, "Let's take the bus." Robert was incredulous; he hadn't been on a bus for years. In no time, they were at the bus stop and soon sitting on the bus, out of the snow, warming up. After five minutes of viewing Manhattan from the height only afforded by a bus view, Robert said, "This is fun." The image conveys comic relief.

Over the years, Diane has shared powerful stories of Christian Science healings that always give me hope and inspiration. There are so many paths to God. How could there not be when the world is so diverse, and we are all given the freedom to find our own way?

Having Diane's prayers and intervention on my side is a powerful bond. At the end of our visit, I give her all the details I have so far about my disease, and she shares several recent experiences she has had with healings. I ask her to say prayers of healing for me. She is delighted I have asked, and explains she could not say intervening prayers for a healing without my permission. How fascinating—just like the doctors and the HIPAA rule. "By all means you have it," I say. Having this friend and her powerful prayers on my team is a comfort, and the new MOMA is a treat, seeing so many familiar paintings newly hung. I miss seeing the four Henry Moore bas-relief male torsos on the garden wall where they have always been. They have been moved to an inside room—big mistake—but all other changes are for the better.

Diane and I talk about Mallorca at the end of our afternoon. She is delighted to be included in the birthday invitation, but has some conflicts and will not be able to come. We talk about a visit to Spain the following summer. Our departure hug is harder than usual.

As I revert to taxi travel back to the Regency Hotel, I reflect on the many paths to God. I remember as a child growing up in the strictest version of the Catholic faith. You were not supposed to read anything about religion unless it had the stamp of approval of the Catholic Church, the "imprimatur" at the beginning of the book. I know just where the copy of Etienne Gilson's *The Christian Philosophy of St. Thomas Aquinas* is on my bookshelf at home, which, along with a collection of other religious books from college, bears the imprimatur on the first page. We read and studied Aquinas's spin on Christianity far more than the Bible as I moved through the ranks at Catholic schools. I remember being a bridesmaid in a Protestant wedding and having to get a special dispensation from the Catholic Church to participate in a service in a non-Catholic church. Thank goodness these shackles have been lifted. I love the young hero in Yann Martel's *The Life of Pi*, who practices all of the major religions at once, kneeling to Mecca, receiving the Eucharist, observing the Sabbath. I love Bruce Feiler's inclusive Abraham, arguing the same man is the father of all Muslims, Christians, and Jews.

On Tuesday, I take lunch to my glamorous New York friend, Camilla, who has been dealing with "medical challenges" herself and fights daily battles armed with elegance and grace. Camilla is an inspiration as a person who lives life to the fullest, with a very successful jewelry business while fighting gradual deterioration from MS. Again I wonder if I should tell her about my diagnosis and ultimately decide to fess up for the same reason I told Diane. Camilla gives me the name and number of a close friend of hers recovering from leukemia. I thank her, but I'm not ready to swap stories with strangers. I know I am not ready to contact her, just as I am not going to call the leukemia support group number posted in Dr. Greer's office. Just beginning to share my story with close friends is the succor I need right now. Is it a blessing to have the character trait that made me want to share my diagnosis with friends? I wonder, for many others do not want to talk about their illnesses.

We go to Jim's business dinner, the purpose of the trip, at the Trattoria del Arte in the Soho area. I sit next to Lynn, a recent survivor of breast cancer. She is from Nashville and has already heard something was going on with me. "What?" The Nashville grapevine is moving fast. She confides that once you have been diagnosed with cancer (she can say the word—she had it), you move from a line of healthy over to a line of sick for life, no matter how many years a disease is in check. Our conversation continues on a far more intimate level than usual dinner table topics. The cathartic details of her survival make me realize again that I'm not alone. Her perspective, however, gives me pause. "I had a terrible attitude the whole time. I was miserable, sick as a dog. I don't care what people say; I don't think attitude makes any difference in dealing with cancer. You just grit your teeth and get through it and move on." Wait a minute, wasn't it important to assume a positive attitude? Apparently this ingredient was not a part of my friend's recovery. I was baffled. Everyone has the right to choose his or her own path, yet I already knew this would not be mine.

The rest of the time in New York, I cover Madison and Fifth Avenues in mission mode. In Armani, where I usually just feel the lush fabrics, I buy the most expensive pair of shoes in my spending history. I hit Saks Fifth Avenue and try on a Zoran outfit in the designer salon. I've done this before, said I'd think about it and imagined going home and whipping it up on the sewing machine. The outfit is a perfect, off-white jacket in one silk, pants and camisole in another slightly different shade of silk that coordinates subtly with the jacket. Drop-dead gorgeous fabric and simple design, elegant beyond belief. As usual I say, "I'll think about it," and start to take it off as I think of the sewing machine. Then I hear myself say, "Wait a minute." I crack open the door of the dressing room and call the saleslady back. "I'll take it." I feel elated. Maybe I'm sick, but I'm going to look smashing at the summer party in June planned before the diagnosis. Better than wine.

Spiritual Dimension

*I*always love being back in New York and knowing that this exciting place is my hometown. But the three days pass in a flash, and on Wednesday night, we return home. The Zoran outfit is on its way to Nashville, on another plane in the charge-and-ship-out-of-state, no-tax box. I look down on the sunset from our plane. Two-thirds of the sky is a black frame, an outline for slits of yellow light and pink glow and above a sky of vivid, pansy blue, gradually fading to darker hues and finally deep grey. I keep my eye on blue, the color clear enough to take my breath away, until the last color lines fade, disappear. Sunsets from above the clouds by a window provide an orchestra seat for nature's nightly painting. I reach out to cover Jim's hand. Our marriage has crossed thirty-eight years. Tranquility settles in when you hit about thirty. You know you will make it to the end. You know you will experience all family rituals as a team. You know you will share the endings. With the beach and shopping buffer over, I am blessed to have Jim's strength and support as anxiety moves into the space I have tried to fill with distraction and denial.

In bed at last, I toss and turn most of the night. Stomach. No, back. No, stomach. Tomorrow, my drill of testing will begin. I begin to wonder if I will be able to stay in control or if my anxiety will turn into depression.

I know all about depression. I am a student of depression. I just hope I am in the graduate category. In the early '90s, I was diagnosed with clinical depression. With my prescription of Zoloft, I went into therapy, slowly and painfully becoming whole again. I remember days when I wasn't sure I could get out of bed. I remember session after session with my shrink, Gordon, laying my life on the table and then slowly putting back the pieces one chapter at a time. If you ever have one of those "can't get out of bed" days, here's a suggestion: Force yourself, force yourself to think of someone, anyone, for whom you can do something nice. It could be a phone call focused completely on the other person (no talking about self allowed). It could be a book shared, a batch of cookies delivered. Once you do this, you have gotten out of the self-focused funk and taken a tiny step. toward recovery. It worked for me. I file this away knowing it might be helpful in the days ahead.

When I first met with my therapist, Gordon, who was also an Episcopal priest, I asked how long this therapy stuff was going to take. He said, "Quite a while." "How long is quite a while?" "Sometimes five or six years." "Five or six years?" I remember going home and thinking about how I had rambled uncontrollably during our first session. I needed to be more organized. I wasn't going to ramble for five years. I was also determined to keep honesty and a positive spin part of the process. I was angry. Mad as hell. Ready to kill. I remember thinking if I opened my mouth to voice all the negative things, a parade of snakes and lizards would come out and I would never be able to control them, never be able to take back the venom they spread. How could I keep a positive spin on what I needed, desperately needed to vent? And now, as I feel anger again building up with each change of my cancer status, I wonder if I will be able to keep it under control. I must remember what I learned when I was going through therapy. The key to controlling my anger was to journal, to write it out, to put the anger on paper and give it a positive spin.

I remember that after my mother died in the late '80s, the burden of painful memories was too heavy to process. My mother didn't just commit suicide; she jumped off the top of the five-story apartment building in Nashville where she and my father had been living for less than a year. I had talked them into retiring to Nashville when they were too old to live in their house in North Carolina. The plan was a disaster for my mother, and the grief from her death paralyzed me. I was stuck for years in a frozen state. The only way I could deal with my mother's sudden flight off the top of a building was to create a large enough room in the back of my brain for the oversized duffel bags filled with unresolved issues, push them inside and close the door very tightly. Over the years, other issues just stacked up on top of those, also remaining in the darkest recesses of my mind, until the pile was so heavy that I knew it could crash on top of me if I disturbed it in any way. As the pile grew, my anger grew. Two years of therapy were needed to unravel the mess.

There is a Southern truism that a girl doesn't become a woman until her mother dies. It took another three years (until my father's death in 1993) for me to begin to become that woman, taking the time through therapy to pay attention first, to the loss of my father, the only person who would ever love me unconditionally. The loss was a deep wound, but also became the celebration of an incredible life. My therapeutic journaling started with stories about my father. Somehow, in addressing that loss, I finally unstuck enough to address other unresolved issues as well. The first story I read to Gordon was about my father.

I would sit down at the computer in my home office and write out each subject I wanted to discuss: my Catholic childhood, the fears of the unfulfilled dreams that would never be part of my reality, the void left by the death of my father, my frustrations with Jim regarding money (I'm the spender). I saved the fears of becoming my mother with all her frailties for last. As I wrote, I would ask God to stick around and help me to be honest and open and write with a positive spin. The next week, I would take the pages in and read them to Gordon.

I remember walking with Nicky after the second session. She asked me how it was going. "I read him my story." "You read him a story?" "Hell, it's my fifty-minute hour, I can do whatever I want." As I wrote, I learned that the anger I was feeling towards everyone around me was really the anger inside of me. I was mad at myself and taking it out on the people close by. As I talked, I began to learn who I was under the shell. I learned to pay attention to the questions below the surface. I learned by writing down the complicated parts of my life, the things too painful to verbalize, I clarified issues one at a time and cut the therapy time down to two years with positive resolution. Sometimes I think of the two years in therapy in my mid-forties as the time I finally became an adult. I worked so hard during those two years. I hope the lessons I learned could serve me now. As my equilibrium begins to shatter once again, I must hold on to those lessons, and I must again ask God to sit on my shoulder.

God was an old friend. I was grounded in childhood with a strong spiritual base. I grew up on the campus of Manhattanville College, the all-women's Catholic college where my father taught classics and archeology. The college was run by the Religious of the Sacred Heart nuns. When my brother and I were little, the college was in New York City and we lived in the village. I love to tell people, "I was born in Greenwich Village." I love to think that somehow the aura of New York is a permanent stamp on my personality. I never outgrew New York, but the college did, and in the early '50s the campus moved to 150 beautiful acres in the then rural area of Purchase, New York, forty miles outside the city. The nuns lived in the cloister in the upstairs of the original stone mansion on the estate, and were like a large congregation of aunts. We lived in one of the houses on the estate. I went to the nearest convent school run by the same order in Greenwich, Connecticut, for grammar school and high school, and then I went to Manhattanville for college. I lived in the dorm during college, and before each vacation, some clever student would ask if I had my airline reservations yet. My friends loved walking over to my parents' house in the evening for cocktail hour. Technically, drinking was verboten on the campus. Shoot, as freshmen, we even had a lights-out policy at 10:00 PM. We pretended our house on the edge of the property didn't count as part of the campus. In my parents' living room, debates were lively and topics ranged from politics to history to campus concerns. My father's historical perspective always added a level of reflection to the topic. We never mentioned our off-campus outings to the nuns. Years later Jim would say, "Those nuns really messed with your head." But I didn't feel stifled or over-whelmed as Jim imagined; to the contrary, I felt stimulated and challenged. For me, the nuns represented the most sophisticated teaching of the Catholic Church. And their teaching stuck to me like glue. Even though I rolled my eyes with the best of them over ridiculous rules imposed over the years by overzealous nuns, I graduated from college with a generally positive attitude towards my schooling, a deep and enriching faith, and a great admiration for the women who were my mentors.

Then I married and moved to Nashville and could not find a comfortable place to practice my faith. The Catholic Church here was primitive in comparison to my former experience. The sermons on Sundays focused on hell flavored with guilt, and I would come home angry rather than inspired. Jim isn't Catholic and did not share my history. How could I ever entice him to attend these services with any regularity? I tried Catholic churches in various parts of Nashville, but failed to feel a connection, or even a fleeting glimpse of the rituals of my past. When Jamie was born, I found a bright, young Catholic priest who performed his baptism. By the time Daniel was ready to be baptized, the young priest had left the priesthood to get married. I took it as a sign. I needed to make a change, too. Several good friends attended the same Episcopal church as Jim's parents and suggested that it would be easier to encourage Jim to attend the same church where his father was still on the vestry. The decision was so difficult for me that I went to one of my "aunty" nuns at Manhattanville and laid the problem at her feet. In tears I asked, "How can I practice my faith in a place where it doesn't exist?" She said, "Imagine if you had moved to England. That doesn't mean that you would have to give up your American citizenship. But as long as you were in England, you would need to live by their customs." That made sense. As long as I was in Nashville, I would find another solution for our family. I went home, and we started to attend the Episcopal church just a few blocks from our house.

There was only one problem. I couldn't join. I was a Catholic. So for the twenty or so years our boys were growing up, I attended that Episcopal church but never joined the congregation. What's more, I could not really pray in that foreign atmosphere. For twenty years, my spiritual growth was on hold. As I look back, my inability to move on seems absurd, but beliefs embedded in a Catholic education spanning from early childhood through college are not lightly shed. As a child, I was taught I was blessed to be chosen to receive the unique Sacred Heart education in the one, holy, Catholic and

Apostolic Church, and I was expected to wear the privilege through life like a holy mantle, passing on my gift to my children and their children. Funny how many churches claim to be the one, true Church. Only when I was going through therapy in the early '90s, when I took the time to really ask God to help me make a decision for myself, did I find my new spiritual home in another Episcopal church, Christ Church Cathedral in downtown Nashville. And even with the therapy, it wasn't easy. God had to talk to me directly. He had to get in my face and tell me it was OK to practice my faith in an Episcopal church. He had to assure me He was there, too, before I believed it. As my comfort level grew in the safe haven of my new downtown spiritual home, I could hear Him assure me I was not my mother after all. I hold enough of my father to beat another depression and retain my spiritual core.

But for the first time since my early '90s struggles, I am shaky again. I often wonder how much of keeping my faith in a holding pattern for twenty years was the cause of my earlier depression. In a notebook of favorite inspirational readings, I found an old sermon of Gordon's from when he was a priest at Christ Church. It had a quote from Eugene O'Neill, "Man is born broken. He lives by mending. The grace of God is glue." For years I yearned for the close connection I felt as a child when, occasionally, I was touched by the weekly ritual of Sunday Mass, when everything was in sync, like the perfect sunset, and I would feel a brief opening into a powerful spiritual source. Those glimpses sustained me, allowed me to hold onto a thread of the mystery passing through me before moving on to the next person in need. I thank God for my renewed spiritual base, my home at Christ Church Cathedral, my close access to the "glue," as anxiety tries to carve a new crater in the pit of my stomach.

I am still tossing and turning, but I am thankful to be in a better place than I had once been. As I reflect back on dealing with my parents' deaths, I wish I had been able to be more attentive to both events at the time. But perhaps the knowledge I took away from both passings is greater than I thought. Now I am familiar enough with death to look at the possibility of my own in the eye and pay better attention. Maybe I will also learn to do a better job with friends who suffer serious illnesses. The South is attentive and well-versed in how to rally to the call when death visits someone we know. As soon as someone, anyone we slightly know, dies, the news spreads like a forest fire during a drought. In our close community with an unusually wide circle of friends, death visits too often to be ignored. We are forced to think about death and spread news of death in the "did you hear?" category, but my observation is that we also keep a distance. We will think about it tomorrow, unless it hits us in the face; a little later, unless it's our spouse or our child; let's wait a bit. Yes, of course, I'm interested, but not now.

At the moment I am preoccupied with the rhythms of life and death. I can't stop thinking about rituals. Do rituals hold the key to a healthy life? Not just the sacred rituals we perform in church, but perhaps even our ordinary rituals—my rituals—of getting up in the morning, reaching for the brown, cone-shaped coffee filter, measuring the Starbucks decaf coffee, listening to the perking, smelling the aroma, pouring the brew into my favorite pottery mug, adding just the right amount of 1% milk. Or Christmas morning and Jim's yule log for the fire and the *Messiah* music and the stuffed stockings I have needlepointed for the boys and then for Lisa and then for Jack and now Baker's stocking, still in my mind. I think Baker's stocking will have an angel. How many times do I need to repeat these tasks before they speak to my heart? Why is this repetition, whether of the celebration of the Eucharist or the cup of morning coffee, so important? Is it the repetition that awakens our mind to a higher level of consciousness?

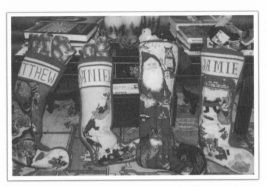

Christmas stockings.

Jim's goddaughter, Lissa, a kindred spirit, gave me a small book, a reprinted lecture on spirituality, *The Quotidian Mysteries, Laundry, Liturgy and "Woman's Work"* by Kathleen Norris. As I grapple with the importance of ritual, I pick up this little book. I keep thinking, yes, yes. The author talks about the cyclical quality in creation: morning and night, the work week and the Sabbath, the earth revolving around the sun, and the seasons. So much of what God has created is repeated yearly, weekly, daily, over and over, like laundry and liturgy and "woman's work." "God's attention is indeed fixed on the little things," making life accessible to us and patterns repeated and giving us the chance to get it right. We may choose to see drudgery, or an opportunity for the sacred. I imagine my life slowing down and see myself at home, in bed, recovering from a series of treatments. I have learned that you have chemo, feel like hell, begin to recover and feel like yourself, and then return for the next cycle of bad and then better. A repetition occurring every three weeks.

Maybe staying away from depression is just showing up with attentiveness to the rhythms of life, adding ritual to the ordinary, until we get it right. I will need ritual, at home and at church and at the hospital, to survive the next step. Finally, in spite of myself, I fall asleep.

Various Extractions

The next day, Thursday, April 21, round B of the medical marathon begins. Anne and Connie take me back to Vanderbilt for an early morning seven-thirty appointment in Dr. Greer's office for a bone-marrow needle biopsy. Jim is in Chicago on business. I also have an afternoon appointment today and a second biopsy tomorrow. Instructions are issued for another empty-stomach arrival for the following day's biopsy. Surely I will lose weight. I have read in the CLL literature given to me on my last visit and additionally on the Internet site describing CLL that weight loss could be one of the symptoms. A cancer perk, please. Dr. Greer's nurse practitioner, Ellen, administers the test. I have been told they could administer a local pain shot or they could put me under in a twilight sleep. The procedure will be painful, and my hip will feel as if I have fallen hard on a sheet of ice. Are you kidding? I go for the twilight sleep, extra dose if available. More please. I feel nothing, remember nothing, and go home where I sleep with the lowest level of consciousness since the diagnosis. I needed that twilight sleep. When I awake, the area on my backside where the needle entered is sore (and will be for a few days), but it is only a slight discomfort, no sense of having fallen on hard ice. Why do the nurses predict the worst?

I realize that my partners Connie and Anne stayed at the house to watch over me only when they wake me up for the next appointment at one-thirty. The three of us go back to Vanderbilt for a pre-op meeting with Dr. Kelly, who will do the full-lymph biopsy the next day. Anne and Connie come in for the consult. After years together with our antiques business, the three of us have fine-tuned the art of collective consulting and decision making. I have quickly learned that in order to digest any new medical lingo, a scribe is essential and two are even better. Dr. Kelly examines under my arms and asks on what side I would like the biopsy. I register shock. Why wouldn't they automatically invade the bad side? How could the smaller lump on the right show the same thing? In the end, rather than taking a single node from the right, we decide to take a few nodes stuck together by the nature of the disease on the left, even though Dr. Kelly explains that the multiple removal will be a more invasive surgery. This will serve to reduce the size of the left lump, and I will be more comfortable if chemo is not deemed necessary. With the various diagnoses, I reason that the chance still exists that a course of "watchful waiting" is a possibility. I don't want to live with that big lump. Out with it.

I listen again to the explanation that a blood cancer like leukemia is systemic, that the cancer exists throughout your blood stream. The tumor cannot be isolated and removed in the way that breast cancer or another type of cancer can because it is not localized, not contained. I listen, but I still don't understand how a biopsy from the other side could be as effective. I do have a decidedly large lump.

At home that night, I give Jim the plan. From his research reading, he lists possible consequences of multiple lump removal and the latter problems of lymphodema: arms swelling and losing mobility, both possible side effects from early overtreatment. He can't understand why they need to take more than one node. He furrows his brow in the way I hate, and his voice takes on an edge as he repeats the question, "Why would they need more than one node for a diagnosis?" Our voices increase in volume, louder in unmonitored space. And I thought it was just maturity when we kept our voices low the other night on the plane, but give me a break. If Jim wants to change the plan, he should have been at the doctor's office. Connie, Anne, and I had made a decision, and the operation is scheduled for six-thirty in the morning. Time has passed for second guessing.

I need affirmation for my decision, and I make my first call to Dr. Greer. He returns the call in short order. Thank you. He concurs with Dr. Kelly and the ladies' decision and that settles it. I call Dr. Roy, who agrees with Dr. Greer. Each step in dealing with cancer seems to involve dancing between the removal of bad cells and the possible disturbance of the good ones. Each step means listening to a series of doctors with a series of suggestions and at the right moment, picking one.

On Friday morning at six-thirty, my empty stomach and I arrive at the Vanderbilt Medical Center East for the lymph-node biopsy, an operation with a sizable cut and a drain left in for the next week. Jim is in attendance for this round. Again I am lost to twilight sleep and then go home to bed for the rest of the weekend, on pain pills, trying to find a position where sleep lasts more than an hour. We are scheduled to attend a charity function on Saturday night. We cancel the first of many public outings. Nesting at home and naps become my daily routine . . . or is it a ritual?

On Sunday morning, I open the door of our bedroom, step onto the side porch, and sink into the wicker sofa. In late April, the garden pulses with new life. The ground is changing from brown to green as leaves of perennials push through the dirt and form variously shaped clusters, spiky iris, puffy nigella. The clumps of peony leaves have expanded from their early spring, wine-colored shoots to their mature, five-fingered shape and dominate the beds like green umbrellas with tiny buds randomly sticking out of the tops. The anticipation of future blooms is like a new birth. The endless possibilities hold no flaw, only promise of beauty to come. The first blooms in cool spring days last

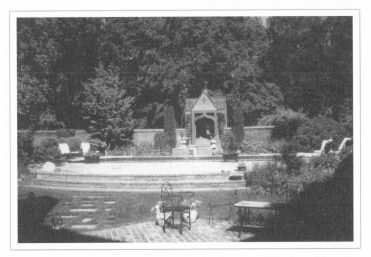

The garden surrounding the pool in spring.

three times longer than later flowers. I find myself in accelerated focus, dreaming of those first peonies when I will fill my favorite pink luster jug with water, adding the blooms one at a time, and then wiping off any moisture left on the bottom of the jug before setting it on wood. The early peonies seem to arrange themselves, the sturdy stems holding the large blooms upright with ease, one flower touching the next until the vase is full. I will place them, as I always do, on Jim's grandmother's Pembroke table by the living room window.

As I think of the peonies, I remember the peony bed in our garden in Purchase and my father weeding on Saturday afternoons. Our house, on an outside corner of the Manhattanville property, had been the gardener's cottage. The variety and choice of plant materials still reflected a studied eye in the years we lived there. My love for gardening came from the landscaped acre around my childhood home. The rhododendron bushes were twenty feet high, the azaleas ten. Across from our driveway was a four-acre apple orchard. The memory of my mother's pies, made from tart, green apples, still makes my mouth water.

In another week, sixty peonies will burst open in my Nashville garden, lush powder puffs, whites, a few with just a blush of pink, next to the blue silla, next to the blue pansies, next to the blue Japanese irises. I love the early spring when the garden opens with just blues and whites and greens. Nothing compares to the beauty and smell of the peonies, yet no flower passes so quickly into oblivion—so pay attention.

Sunday night, Jamie and Lisa and Jack and Baker come over for order-out supper. I am frustrated because my sore arm won't allow me to hold Baker, so Lisa puts her on the bed and we talk nonsense for several glorious minutes. My new granddaughter, the first girl in the Cheek family in four generations, suddenly smiles, her first smile, her very first, rosebud smile, the best flowering of all.

At eight on Monday morning, Nicky and Dana, my next team, take me for a MUGA (Multiple Gated Acquisition) scan and a CAT scan, back in the radiology department behind the front entrance to the hospital. The MUGA scan measures the rate at which the blood flows from the heart back to the body. A strong heart is a necessary prerequisite for chemo. The CAT scan is a sophisticated x-ray dissecting the body into cross sections. We sit in the waiting room until I am called into the scan room where the test will take place. I sit on a metal table as a preoccupied technician tells me they will draw blood, mix it with radioactive material, and put it back in my vein. Then I'll drink some liquid that tastes like chalk and wait for half an hour.

"Do you want an IV or a butterfly stick?"

"What?"

"The IV will be a one-time stick, the needle taped to your left hand and reused when I put the blood back in. The prick would be two times, once for the initial blood and again when I put the blood back."

I have been in control until this moment, able to handle each step in this unfolding drama with me in the starring role. But I have just hit information overload. The number of times I would be stuck by a needle over the next month flashes into my brain and I lose it. I try to focus on the floor as tears stream down my cheeks. The technician softens into a real person before my eyes. "You're new at this?" she says. I ask, "What would you choose?" "I hate IVs, I'd go for the butterfly." I eke out, "OK." She pricks me once and takes a good sampling. I sit and wait, trying to get some control. When I'm finished and stand up to leave, the technician says, "Do you need a hug?" I nod, she embraces me, gives me the stuff to drink, and sends me back to sit with my friends for the half-hour wait. Although the liquid is described again as chalk-like and difficult to swallow, I find it isn't that bad. Why is the hospital staff adding drama? Do most people need the worst-case scenario? Why?

As the chalky dye works its way into the nooks and crannies of my innards, Nicky, Dana, and I pass the time laughing about a series of family trips we took each New Year's when our kids were in high school: St. Croix, Abaco, a different island each year. I would always bring the leftover Stilton cheese from our Christmas Eve party. The kids would roll their eyes over pasta with Stilton, soup with Stilton, salad with Stilton, every year with Stilton. I wasn't going to waste that delicious wheel of Stilton.

The technician takes me back to the CAT scan room and reinserts the altered blood. I begin to judge the technician's skills by how tightly she wraps the tourniquet. If she wraps the rubber over my shirt and keeps it flat, the pain is far less severe than if directly applied to the skin with the tourniquet twisted into a thin cord. I lie down on the machine, and the CAT cylinder passes over my body and back for about five minutes. I can feel the cool liquid entering and spreading though my vascular system. When the liquid hits my groin, I feel additional loss of control. I have been told the sensation would feel as if I am relieving myself, and this time the description is accurate.

Jim Meets Dr. Greer

Tuesday, April 26, two and a half weeks after the initial diagnosis, is my second meeting with Dr. Greer, scheduled for the afternoon. Tuesday is also my regular bridge day. I tell Susie I really want to play. Susie is the first friend I made when I moved to Nashville, and she is Jamie's godmother. I met her at a luncheon my first year in the South, and we clicked immediately. I was still in culture shock and she had just graduated from Smith and understood Yankees. She included me in gatherings with her old Nashville friends. I don't think I ever told her how special those invitations were and how much they were responsible for giving me a sense of belonging for the first time.

As I talk to Susie about the bridge game, we both realize we are short one player. Instead of canceling, she invites a small group of friends who are in the loop about my condition over to her house for lunch. She uses her good china. We sit in the dining room and we eat party food as I fill them in on the past few days. I have been up half the previous night thinking about the meeting with Dr. Greer. Tired but invigorated by the loving vibes of the group, I am off again to his office.

Jim, coming from his office downtown, meets me at 3:15 PM in the Vanderbilt University Medical Center parking lot. We walk to the hematology department for meeting two with Dr. Greer. I go over the cancer terminology in my mind. The CLL is an indolent, low-grade process—no that's not right—it's not a process, it's a malignancy. My left arm is sore as hell, and the wound is talking to me. I must remember to tell Dr. Greer that my bug bites still itch. I must remember to tell him I have used Lamisil for three months on a toe fungus that has now turned into a painful ingrown toenail. That hurts, too. I should mention this, shouldn't I? The podiatrist wants to cut off the ingrown nail, but needs guidance from my oncologists because of the possibility of excessive bleeding after chemo. A week ago, the state of my toes seemed important. And shouldn't he know that I'm overdue for a mammogram? And that I'm overdue to have my teeth cleaned and checked? I remember something about the mouth being the part of the body that is most subject to infection. Since Jim's hip replacement four years ago, he needs to take an antibiotic every time his teeth are cleaned. One of my molars aches. I'm a mess. I clutch my journal, a black marble composition note-book that is becoming a security blanket. I look over the written list of questions as we wait for the door to open.

I introduce Jim to Dr. Greer, who repeats the information he gave us over the phone and then focuses on two concerns: They have found larger cells than usually expected with a diagnosis of CLL, and the #CD 38 marker in the leukemia cell from the bone-marrow biopsy is a concern. On the Rai stage scale of CLL, I have a stage 1 cancer. I hear every word. The new information, the foreign medical language, the reality that I am the patient, that I am the focus of this indecipherable jargon—all are entering my brain but hold little meaning and leave no room for the energy to cover my list of suddenly superficial questions.

The worst frustration is that no results have come from the lab regarding the lymph-node biopsy. I was up half the night wondering, and there is insufficient data to discuss the next procedure. I want to be in the room with Dr. Greer and Jim to lay out the next step. I want to eyeball my doctor and leave here with a secure game plan. Now this important decision in my treatment will be given over the telephone. Dr. Greer mentions the possibility of Richter's syndrome, but that I have none of the usual symptoms. He is reluctant to give a final diagnosis until all the tests are back. He will consult with doctors at M. D. Anderson, at Sloan Kettering, and at Mayo. Dr. Greer outlines on paper possible options from "watchful waiting" to three alternatives of a medium-level chemo, an aggressive chemo, and as a last resort, a stem-cell transplant. His guess would be the medium chemo with fludarabine.

With every change in diagnosis I should be thinking about my health, but I'm thinking about my hair. "Will I lose my hair?" I ask. "Maybe not." He replies. Dr. Greer asks if I have any siblings who could be tested for a match if we need to do a stem-cell transplant. I tell him about my only brother, who lives in Spain. A flash of me diving into the Mediterranean, emerging with slicked-back hair, passes through me and disappears. "Would he need to fly over here?" "He could probably go to a lab in Spain to extract the appropriate blood samples. The problem will be getting the samples here." The challenges of acquiring blood samples from overseas are left hanging.

Dr. Greer goes on to say that the CAT scan shows a slight shadow on the left breast. I need to schedule a mammogram next week. Great. Terrific. At least I can scratch that one off my list of questions. Dr. Greer schedules more tests: a follow-up with Dr. Kelly after the lymph surgery, the mammogram, and an MRI. He says that I need to have any other medical concerns taken care of now, so the toe and the teeth can be scratched off the question list as well, and we can meet in another week to finalize the decisions about my treatment.

I talk to the hospital scheduler—her name is Michele and I now recognize her voice on the phone—about the additional tests. She tells me the MRI will take about half an hour, but to allow an hour and a half. Welcome to hospital time.

I need to get my toe looked at and my teeth cleaned. Dr. Greer has confirmed that anything that might cause bleeding needs to be attended to before starting chemo. I was right—the mouth is especially susceptible to excess bleeding and bacteria growth. I have a gum disease. I forget the name. I'm supposed to have my teeth cleaned every four months. It's been eight. A left, back molar is sensitive. We won't talk about that just yet, but my record for infrequent doctors' visits has self-destructed.

On April 27, I go to the basement of Baptist Hospital to retrieve my old mammogram records so they can be added to future tests at Vanderbilt for comparison purposes. A large, windowless room the size of a concert hall is fitted with floor-to-ceiling rolling, oversized files to accommodate millions of old mammograms. People have to work down there, every day, in the spring, when the sky is an intense blue. I hope the cafeteria these folks use has a window.

Creating a Contact Group

∽

*T*he last weekend of April, we are off on another trip to Ponte Vedra, a trip scheduled before my diagnosis. Jim's dad is turning eighty-seven, and we are taking him down to celebrate. I want life to go on. Back in Florida, near the ocean waves, I am calmer. The telephone rarely rings. People leave us alone. I can digest the various stages of the diagnosis with space and the sea. We will meet with Dr. Greer again on May 4, almost a month from the original diagnosis. I am ready for all test results to be in and a plan finalized.

Before we leave for Florida, I ask Linda to come over and help me compose an e-mail contact list. The information about my disease seems to continually change. I have tried to stay current with my friends, but I am running out of the energy for phone calls, and I will have less when and if treatment starts. I find that once I discuss the latest information with one person on the phone, I have no energy for a repeat performance. Rumors are beginning to circulate, from the worst scenario of Richter's to the most benign version of CLL. I need to calm the fires. Besides, I like e-mail. I am comfortable with the efficiency of the e-mail world, with communicating through the touch of fingers clicking across the keyboard, and the Send command efficiently passing the message into cyberspace.

I am skeptical, scared really, to write about my own illness, but I trust Linda. "Would it be weird, self-serving, strange, if I set up a contact list and wrote to people about myself? I recall receiving e-mails from spouses or family members of friends who are ill but I can't recall a patient who has ever initiated the dialogue. Can I do that?" "Absolutely, you need to do what makes you comfortable," she replies.

Linda's grandson Charlie was diagnosed with cancer at ten months of age. He is healthy now, thank God. Her family developed an amazing e-mail list called "Charlie's Angels" during his illness. Each time he went for treatment, we knew when to send up petitioning prayers, we knew the results of the tests, we could follow the progress and send encouraging words without invading the family space. Charlie's Angel's grew into a powerful support group for Linda's family and their many friends.

Linda and I search the Help menu in Outlook, my e-mail software program, and she clicks on the right buttons. We brainstorm together to come up with a short list of my closest friends made over thirty-seven years in Nashville, the people I want to keep abreast of each change, each decision, and each procedure. I realize how lucky I am that longevity in one place creates a substantial list of close, lifelong friends. We start with eighteen names and send out a short first message:

APRIL 27, 2005

DEAR WONDERFUL FRIENDS,

I HAVE JUST CREATED A GROUP E-MAIL, WITH LINDA'S HELP, AND WANTED ALL OF YOU TO KNOW HOW GRATEFUL I AM FOR ALL OF YOUR WARM WORDS AND PRAYERS. I STILL DO NOT KNOW ALL OF THE RESULTS OF ALL OF ONGOING TESTS THAT HAVE BEEN DONE IN THE PAST WEEKS. I HAVE DEFINITELY BEEN DIAGNOSED WITH CLL, CHRONIC LYMPHOCYTIC LEUKEMIA. I HAD TO LOOK THAT UP TO GET THE SPELLING RIGHT. THIS IS GOOD NEWS, IF YOU HAVE TO HAVE CANCER. PEOPLE LIVE FOR TWENTY PLUS YEARS WITH NO TREAT-MENT. THE RESULTS OF ONGOING TESTS WILL DETERMINE THE PROGRESS OF THE DISEASE.

The next day Linda comes by with a three-ring notebook with
tabs for doctors' visits, phone consultations, list of meds, treatment
schedules, test results, phone numbers of doctors and nurses, and
insurance information. She follows with an e-mail to me:

. . . THE DOCTOR AT SLOAN KETTERING TOLD US THAT WE WERE
ULTIMATELY RESPONSIBLE FOR MAKING SURE THAT CHARLIE WAS
TAKEN CARE OF. BY THAT HE MEANT THAT WE NEEDED TO CHECK
EVERY MEDICATION, EVERY CHEMO DRUG FOR THE NAME AND THE
AMOUNT BEING GIVEN, EVERY TYPE OF ANESTHESIA HE WAS GIVEN,
EVERY INJECTION, ETC. WITH THE NURSE OR DOCTOR WHO WAS
GIVING IT. HIS DOCTOR SAID THAT NO ONE WOULD BE OFFENDED
WHEN ASKED THIS INFORMATION BECAUSE MISTAKES CAN HAPPEN
AND THEY CAN ALSO BE AVOIDED IF YOU ARE DILIGENT.

I had no idea at the time how valuable this information would be.
The focus of the Ponte Vedra weekend is a sunset, birthday
dinner on the terrace of Cap's, our favorite restaurant on the inter-
costal waterway. My stomach is not accepting much sustenance. My
responses to questions are monosyllabic as I try to swallow the lump
in the middle of my throat. I want to go home, go to sleep, feel relief
from this perpetual state of anxiety, and be able to do anything,
anything to turn it off. Jim is being solicitous of Grandpa, working
back and forth between his two favorite subjects, World War II and
science fiction. Grandpa is frail of body, but his mind is as sharp as
steel. Still, we would prefer not to tell him, at eighty-seven, about
my diagnosis, but fear he will hear about it from someone at church
or at the retirement community where he lives. We give him the

bare facts, but it is still information overload. His reaction is denial—not his precious daughter-in-law. He changes the subject and never brings it up again.

We order hors d'oeuvres. I munch at a third of my seafood pasta. Dr. Greer had answered "no" to my last weight-loss inquiry. "You might gain weight with the steroids you will have to take after each chemo." I'd show him. Back at our beach nest, I go to the bedroom and start *The Birdcage*, but even watching Nathan Lane in stockings and skull cap fails to make me react. I take an Ambien and by eight-thirty, I'm asleep.

Back in Nashville on Monday, Nicky and I go for my mammogram across the street from Vanderbilt in another clinic. Of course, I will have to wait for the doctor's reading to hear a report. More waiting.

I go back to the class I have been taking for about five years with Ken, the dean and head priest at Christ Church Cathedral. Raised as a Roman Catholic, my knowledge of the Bible is in the basement, and other classes I have tried over the years didn't reach me. There are endless opportunities for Bible study in Bible Belt country. Ken's class is different. Steeped in fascinating details of the history of the time, the setting in which Christ lived, and the players who surrounded Him, Ken makes the Bible relevant to our daily lives. We spend about three years on any given book of the New Testament. Often a whole class is devoted to a single line. Ken loves to go off on a historical reference or the exact meaning of an original Greek word to delve into a deeper interpretation of the text, and his terrible maps provide comic relief. Many people have been in the class as long as I have, and I feel a connection to the forty or so who form a circle behind thin tables that circumvent the lecture hall behind the sanctuary of the church. Ken verbally welcomes me back. I have missed four weekly classes. I am touched. Currently we are studying the Gospel of John. I am only half there, but I do remember Ken discussing one of my favorite passages, "When two or more are gathered in my name I am with you." He goes on to suggest that Jesus is present in a different way when we are in a group collectively thinking about Him. And I wonder, any time two or more people are together talking about God, is it a prayer?

After class, Kendall, Margo, Anne Taylor, Eugenia, Coleman, Virginia, and Judy all gather around me to say they have been thinking about me and praying for me. They know I am sick because I have been on the church prayer list. I knew I was on the list, but this is my first experience of connection to my fellow Christ Church family.

I didn't make a call to the church and ask to be put on the prayer list. In fact, I told Ken I wasn't ready to have my name read outloud at each church service: how embarrassing, how self-serving, calling undue attention to myself. I wasn't that important. Then I find out Anne had called and asked to have me put on the list, and it slips by Ken. Fortunately, I was not in the church the first Sunday my name was read. I would have melted under the seat. But then I start getting notes and phone calls from church members. One couple whom I barely know sends a note with one line, "You are in our thoughts and prayers," every other week for months. People see me and ask how I am doing. Instead of embarrassed, I begin to feel surrounded by an overwhelming, nurturing blanket, soft and warm. Today, returning to class, people know I am sick and shower me with their concerns.

The group surrounding me after class stays for an unusual amount of time. Stories of healing are passed around. I know, even though we never speak of these issues, that these women are spiritually grounded, even spiritually connected with me, having shared this class over a span of years. Suddenly I feel free to share my preoccupation with what it means to pray, how different it is to be the recipient of prayer, and how I am trying to wrap my mind around the idea. One has a sister who had lymphoma ten years ago, and we hear a brief summary of her remarkable recovery. One has a son with chronic allergies, and she never knows if the next call will be the school with a problem. She has lived with fear for fourteen years. Both speak to me about the comfort of prayer. One suggests praying together, perhaps in my garden. My friends want to hear about my illness, want details of the diagnosis. We are all exploring, talking together about questions usually left in the silence of our minds. In the safety of a loving connection, the power is immeasurable. Rolling over and over in my mind is the thought that this moment shared is a prayer, and Jesus is here with us as we gather in our honest struggles toward collective truth. For the first time, I witness the power of community and the gift of embracing like-minded pilgrims on the same road, with the presence of these amazing women easing my way.

They recommend two books on dealing with illness and death as we part, Marianne Williamson's *A Return to Love* and Bernie Siegel's *Love, Medicine and Miracles*. They are the first of many books recommended or given to me over the coming months. I buy them on the way home. They are OK. Over time, I will receive or hear about dozens of books to help understand the struggle I will endure. My hands-down favorite is written by four women from Nashville, *Speak the Language of Healing: Living with Breast Cancer without Going to War*, by Carol Matzkin Orsborn, Linda Quigley, Karen Leigh Stroup, and Susan Kuner. They all had breast cancer and answer the same series of well-posed questions about living with cancer with candor and empathy and soul.

After class, Anne Taylor and I walk to the Frist Center Art Museum, across the street in the restored deco post office, for lunch and continued conversation. Our friendship bonded over writing about ten years ago. When I first started to write, I asked her, a creative writing teacher, if I could pay her to help me with my rusty skills. She thought about it for a few days and called back to say that as a poet, she would like a prose writer to critique her poetry. Why didn't we just get together as friends and critique each other? As so often happens in midlife, a mutual pursuit blossomed into friendship. We stopped working together a few years back, and now had catching up to do. I was beginning to notice a willingness among many friends to slow down as I slowed down, and to enjoy a quiet moment with me.

The e-mails turn into another way to keep connected. The responses I receive from friends after the first e-mail are affirming. I sense people want to be connected with me in my struggle. I sense bonds forming. I find the second message easier to write even though what I have to say is more difficult. I need to tell my new team that the diagnosis for Richter's syndrome is confirmed. The decision to start chemo is confirmed. I want them to hear this from me, and I want to keep the tone upbeat. I sense that, as with my early writing during therapy, I need to send messages with a positive spin.

UPDATE FROM PATIENT SIGGY
MAY 2, 2005
DEAR WONDERFUL FRIENDS,

I WANT TO SHARE WITH YOU ANOTHER UPDATE FROM MY ONCOLOGIST, JOHN GREER, MD. BY THE WAY, BOTH DR. ROY AND DR. JOHN TOLD ME THAT IF THEY HAD THIS PROBLEM, DR. GREER WOULD BE THEIR FIRST CHOICE OF PHYSICIAN.

DR. GREER CALLED US IN FLORIDA ON FRIDAY WITH THE UNFORTUNATE REPORT THAT THE FULL-LYMPH BIOPSY CONFIRMED THE TURNOVER OF LARGE CELLS IN MY LYMPH NODES. I HAVEN'T GOT THE LINGO STRAIGHT YET, BUT THE BOTTOM LINE IS THAT THE DISEASE HAS PROGRESSED FURTHER THAN IS USUALLY FOUND IN AN EARLY DIAGNOSIS OF CLL. THE WORD TO DESCRIBE MY CONDITION IS RICHTER'S SYNDROME OR RICHTER'S TRANSFORMATION—AT

LEAST THIS IS THE DIAGNOSIS OF THE DAY. THE GOOD NEWS IS THAT MY BLOOD IS NORMAL AND THE ONLY SYMPTOMS I HAVE ARE THE ENLARGED LYMPH NODES. I ALSO WENT TO HAVE A MAMMOGRAM TODAY AND IT WAS COMPLETELY CLEAR. HOORAY.

THE BAD NEWS IS THAT I WILL HAVE TO GO THROUGH CHEMO FOR SIX TO EIGHT MONTHS. JIM AND I WILL MEET WITH DR. GREER ON WEDNESDAY AND PROBABLY HEAR THE GAME PLAN. YOU WILL HAVE TO CONTINUE BEING REALLY NICE TO ME FOR THE FORESEE-ABLE FUTURE, SO DEAL WITH IT.

I AM THINKING A LOT ABOUT THE FACT THAT NOW PEOPLE ARE PRAYING FOR ME. WHAT DOES THAT REALLY MEAN? IF I CAN THINK OF A GIFT THAT I HAVE RECEIVED, ALONG WITH ALL OF THESE FRIGHTENING REPORTS, IT IS THAT TODAY IS PRECIOUS AND ALL OF MY FRIENDS ARE A TREASURED SOURCE OF SUPPORT.

THANK YOU FOR YOUR LOVE, FLOWERS, HUGS, AND ESPECIALLY PRAYERS. KEEP THEM COMING.

HUGS, SIGOURNEY

The e-mail list is growing. With the first e-mail, a surprising number of people forward my message to others who e-mail back and asked to be added to the list. My message now goes out to forty-five people.

A lawyer friend, Barbara, reminded me that five years ago e-mails were just hitting their stride in the workplace. Now this speedy communication tool is affecting most of our lives. With this second message I don't go into much detail about the diagnosis, other than to say that my symptoms are atypical for Richter's. I don't want people to be alarmed. I don't want people thinking," Poor Sigourney." Besides, I am having difficulty grappling with the meaning myself. I have a terrible disease with a bad prognosis, yet I have few of the terrible symptoms. I have not had CLL for a long time. I do not have multiple places with enlarged lymph nodes. So does that reverse the bad prognosis? Too much analysis will drive me over the brink.

Garden Party

⌒

I need a distraction. On Tuesday, I switch gears, putting my illness on hold. Tuesday evening we host the first pre-diagnosis planned event that I would not cancel. How can I explain it? As my world turns upside down, my garden is an oasis against change, an acre of normal right outside my bedroom door. I need to maintain some focus outside of illness to survive the journey ahead. A year ago I had agreed to host a dinner, two tables of ten, for a group of people from around the country who would be in Nashville for a meeting of the Garden History and Design Committee of the archives of the Smithsonian Institute. My favorite caterer, Rachel, is on the books to supply dinner. I can set the tables with my best china with my eyes closed. Flower guru Julie is booked to design center-pieces in silver baskets with peonies and roses that everyone will think came from my garden. I have secured my favorite waiter, Freddy, who knows our kitchen better than I do. My gardener, the other Jim, has the beds in showcase form. All I have to do is show up. This is also a payback to my friend, Tooty, who is in charge of the event and has asked me to host this dinner.

Tooty saved my life last year by becoming the "Badge Nazi" for a National Garden Club of America event I chaired. Attending were 150 out-of-towners with assorted titles and multiple and assorted egos. Their badges had to have every "i" dotted, be color-coded, and tied with the right color ribbon so they could hang from necks and not spoil the silk blouses or designer suits with, God forbid, a pin prick. I love the Garden Club and all its rich programs about horticulture, but please. I guess if you had a title that was earned after hundreds of hours of work, you would want it to be right, but my detail-itis does not go in that direction. Tooty spent untold hours combing over the twenty-column spreadsheet, making sure every one of those 150 tags was correct. I would never let Tooty down after what she did for me, even though my close friends are ready to kill me for not canceling tonight's dinner. Besides, I need one more distraction. I need one more focus on my old world, misfocused as it might be at the moment.

My spirits lift as the house transforms for the party. The polished brass threshold at the front door and the fresh flowers throughout the house send a sign that life is still full. I am in control. Jim and I bought our Tudor-style brick house thirty years ago. Built in the 1920s, the house had little maintenance in the twenty years before we took over. The third generation of the original family were elderly and had been neglectful for fifteen years. Another family who lived there for the next five years lacked the money to fix it up and finally put it back on the market. The house had been on the market for over a year with the reputation of an albatross, but to me it had beautiful bones and endless possibilities. We made a low bid and successfully bought into a slow, continuous renovation project for the next several decades.

Right away we gutted the kitchen, ripped out shag carpet, restained floors, painted, and moved in with our three boys, ages five years to six months, with a hot plate and a fridge in the dining room. We were young. The first time I went to the front door, the delivery person asked, "Is your mother home?" During the first weeks of renovation, as I was down on my knees with pliers pulling the nails left from the carpet liner out of the floor, Jim came home and told me we were the laughingstock of Nashville for having bought this house.

Eighteen years ago, we added a serious addition of a midlife-crisis state-of-the-art downstairs master bedroom and bath with an outdoor terrace and extended, walled garden that I look out at and treasure each morning before the start of the day.

Last year a top real-estate agent in town called to say one of his clients wanted only our house and to name a price. Now we can be the ones to laugh and we're not ready to sell.

There was no garden and little landscaping when we bought the house. Over the years, my passion has been the development of an acre of undulating flower beds, the majority set off inside a six-foot, serpentine, brick wall. I was thrilled when our garden was chosen as one of the first in Nashville to be photographed and recorded in the archives of the Smithsonian Institute as part of the Garden Club of America initiative to record special gardens across the country. Now I had the chance to meet and entertain the committee who had made the archives possible. I didn't want to miss it.

I don't attend to all the usual preparty details. The silver picture frames in the living room remain slightly tarnished. The family room and the upstairs bedrooms remain unfluffed. Marcella, another detail queen, is one of many friends who asks what she can do for me after hearing of my diagnosis. Instead of making another casserole, she comes and spends the morning setting the tables with one grand-mother's silver and another grandmother's china and linens. I spend the afternoon in bed.

When Jim comes in at six to change and set up the bar, I break down and start to cry. Don't ask me why I cry, but I wash my face, powder my nose, and the dinner goes off without a hitch. Several guests take clumps of *Adenophora*, a variety of ladybells, back to Delaware and New Jersey. I dug the original clump years ago from a neighbor's garden and have yet to see the specimen offered in any nursery. My level of exhaustion is worth every minute.

And Then More Tests

$\mathcal{T}$he fresh flowers last for a week, but the next day I am back at Vanderbilt for more tests. I go by myself on Wednesday for a post-op visit with Dr. Kelly, who performed the lymph node operation. I circle around the clinic parking garage, stopping often behind a hesitant senior who shouldn't have been behind the wheel. I walk across the road to the huge three-sectioned Henry Joyce Cancer Center waiting room. Almost all the seats are taken. A wide-screen TV dominates the center room. It's unusually cool for the beginning of May, and I wear my favorite soft winter sweater. The hospital is always cold, and the sweater reaches from the top of my neck, down over my rear. I wrap the softness over my tummy and rub my hands across the knitted cables, thinking of grandson Jack and the security blanket he calls his "bee," a foot-square, soft velour cloth with the face of an elephant in one corner. Again I am struck by the diversity around me. A slender, young woman with hair beginning to grow back under a red baseball cap sits in a wheelchair on my right. I don't think that will be my look. On the other side, a pencil-thin senior, no teeth, new jeans, is next to his wife? sister? An African-American woman is a fashion statement in striped jacket and matching pants.

A credenza on the left holds coffee thermoses and an assortment of Krispy Kreme doughnuts and apples delivered free daily to cancer waiting rooms throughout the hospital. I will learn that carts with packaged crackers, cookies, and danish are also wheeled around by volunteers who take care of the patients in the rooms where chemo and radiation treatments are administered.

Of the forty-plus people present, only two are reading newspapers. Only one lady is absorbed in a dog-eared paperback. I notice a bookshelf in one corner with a selection of similar offerings, probably our reader's source. The rest of the crowd just sits, staring straight ahead. I think of the hours spent in silence, waiting. What do people think about when they sit, staring? How many hours will I clock in various Vanderbilt waiting rooms? I will know this afternoon, maybe tomorrow, maybe the next day, the exact chemo treatment that we will use. I will know the exact time the chemo session will last. Sally, another breast-cancer-surviving friend, told me, "The uncertainty of not knowing the facts, not knowing the procedure ahead is the worst. Once you have a game plan, you can embrace it and move forward." I can tell you that the unknowing is a killer.

Between trips to Florida and New York, I have been at Vanderbilt almost every day. I fill out the same forms with each visit: pain choice, mild to moderate to acute; pain scale, 1 to 10. Educational needs met? Medications understood? Nutrition OK? Lost or gained ten pounds? (In my dreams). Has my daily routine changed? Problems with dressing, toiletry, bathing, walking, eating, standing, social environments? No one threatening me, hurting me, am I afraid? Yeah, I'm afraid, sleep-deprived, anxiety-riddled, but I am safe from any bodily harm. I try to imagine the horror of trying to survive cancer and being continuously afraid of bodily harm from a caregiver.

The nurse calls my name. My blood pressure is 160 over 96. I refuse to get on the scale. I am at the hospital almost every day. How many times do I need to be reminded of my weight? On the day of the lymph-node operation, I got on the scale because the nurse needed to know my weight to administer the correct dosage of meds. Now I say, "I'm not doing that," and somehow gain an ounce of control.

I meet with Dr. Kelly, who removes the drain from the lymph-node operation and checks my wound. The nurse gives me exercises to gradually increase the range of motion for my left arm, which I can only lift to shoulder level. She tells me the recovery will be about three months. Any other time, I would be preoccupied and totally focused on the recovery, but considering what I am about to face, additional arm range is not even on my radar screen.

I go home and take the mail to my bedroom and sit on the bed. I read a thank-you note from a friend who had come to visit a week before the diagnosis. She hopes my toe is better. I had been late for lunch with her because I had gone back to my once-a-year pedicure person because my cured-with-Lamisil postfungus toe was curling and turning into a painful, ingrown toenail. I want to call her and say, "Sweetheart, let me tell you how the toe is *so* not the issue." I resist.

The next day Jim and I meet with Dr. Greer. He again confirms the Richter's syndrome and goes on to say that he has conferred with other doctors at M. D. Anderson, Sloan Kettering, and Mayo Clinic as my disease is so atypical. The consensus is that a stronger chemo, CHOP+R, will be the best choice. M. D. Anderson even recommends a stem-cell transplant, but Dr. Greer thinks that would be too aggressive at this point. He hands us a printout from a computer search of the only other patients he could find with my profile: a large-cell non-Hodgkin's lymphoma occurring in patients with previously undiagnosed CLL. It is a study of seven patients in Yugoslavia. Four out of seven achieved a complete response to an aggressive chemo treatment. We could all think about my treatment once more over the weekend, but he wants us to schedule the port insertion for Thursday and the first chemo on Friday. The first procedure will take about eight hours. Eight hours? Dr. Greer tells us I will have four chemo treatments, one every three weeks. I will be retested at that time and, even if the cancer has gone, they will still do two more treatments. If some cancer remains, they will do an additional four treatments for a total of eight. I hear the words, but the conversation doesn't sink in, the information doesn't compute. I go home and sit at the computer. Sharing my story and knowing friends are following each step give me peace of mind, as does adding another twenty-five people to the list.

UPDATE FROM PATIENT SIGGY
MAY 5, 2005
DEAR FRIENDS,

I AM OVERWHELMED WITH BEAUTIFUL NOTES AND FLOWERS AND E-MAILS FROM SO MANY OF YOU. SOME PEOPLE NEED TO DEAL WITH CRISIS WITHIN THE FAMILY, BUT YOU KNOW ME. I FEEL INCREDIBLE POWER FROM THE LOVE OF ALL OF MY FRIENDS. THANK YOU.

JIM AND I MET WITH DR. GREER ON WEDNESDAY AND THE GOOD NEWS IS THAT I AM A VERY ATYPICAL CANDIDATE FOR RICHTER'S SYNDROME. MOST PEOPLE HAVE THIS AFTER HAVING CLL FOR A LONG TIME. MOST PEOPLE ARE VERY SICK WITH MULTIPLE SYMPTOMS. MY BLOOD IS ALMOST NORMAL, MY HEART IS STRONG, AND I FEEL GREAT. ANXIETY DOESN'T COUNT. I JUST WALKED WITH NICKY AND WILL TRY TO WALK EVERY DAY. JIM AND I ARE GOING TO COLORADO FOR THE WEEKEND TO HELP OUR SON MATTHEW SETTLE INTO HIS NEW HOUSE. WE ARE ALL VERY EXCITED ABOUT THIS NEW STEP IN HIS LIFE. I CAN'T WAIT TO FLUFF. THIS WILL ALSO GIVE DR. GREER TIME TO GET A SECOND OPINION ON PATH REPORTS. WE MEET WITH HIM AGAIN NEXT WEDNESDAY AND WILL BEGIN TREATMENT SOON AFTERWARD. ESTIMATED TIME FOR THE FIRST DOSE IS NOT DETERMINED YET, BUT IT WILL BE A FULL DAY.

THINK OF ME HAVING A WONDERFUL TIME WITH OUR PRECIOUS SON.

HUGS, SIGOURNEY

The early e-mails are short and sugar-coated. Am I protecting my friends, or convincing myself that it's not so bad? Maybe I haven't fully absorbed the data, the reality that chemotherapy will start next week and take eight hours.

The responses are immediate and numerous.

My brother, Kevin, writes:

I AM NOT SURE HOW TO INTERPRET THE TECHNICAL JARGON IN YOUR E-MAIL, SINCE ALL OF THE MEDICAL TERMINOLOGY IS CONFUSING. IT IS HARD TO BELIEVE THIS SCIENCE-FICTION-SOUNDING STUFF IS HAPPENING TO MY BABY SISTER! IN ANY CASE, REMEMBER OUR FAMILY IS REALLY TOUGH AND WILL POWER AND POSITIVE THINKING ARE KICK-ASS TOOLS. I WISH I COULD GIVE YOU A BIG, LONG HUG AND LOTS OF KISSES. IMAGINE THAT I AM DOING IT RIGHT NOW.

Donna affirms:

I AM SO RELIEVED TO HEAR FROM YOU AND KNOW THE STORY . . . OR, AT LEAST, PART OF THE STORY.

Becca writes:

I TOO BELIEVE THAT IN A VOLUNTARY COMMUNITY OF FRIENDS PRAYING FOR ONE ANOTHER THE GREATEST WEALTH OF LIFE IS EXPERIENCED.

How right she is. Dozens of friends share tips on nutrition, exercise, and nurturing. People on the contact list send my message to other friends and acquaintances, such as Taylor and Melinda, who write:

I THINK AS WE ALL GET OLDER, WE RELATE WHEN ANOTHER IS FACED WITH A DIFFICULT STRETCH, WE KNOW THAT WE COULD BE RIGHT THERE, AND WE'RE AWARE THAT EACH DAY WE TURN A NEW PAGE, NOT KNOWING WHAT LIFE WILL BRING TO CHALLENGE US.

Wow. This message is from a couple I have always wanted to know better. Cyberspace is opening a new dimension in my life.

A Breckenridge Break

$\mathcal{O}$n Thursday, Jim and I take off for Denver, excited about helping our youngest son, Matthew, move into his first house—my last distraction before chemo. On the way to the airport, Jim receives a call from a good friend, Jack, who heads a large hospital company in Nashville, offering to do anything he can for me. Another top oncologist in the city works for one of their hospitals, and he will make a call to work me in to see him. I think it over and tell Jim I appreciate the offer, but I have chosen my team and am happy with my decision and don't want to complicate the issue with more opinions. On the plane, we read through medical tomes on Richter's syndrome. I remind myself again of my atypical symptoms. I remind myself of Kevin's positive thinking power—I will win, I will be disease free. The tears still come. I am drained. I try to sleep. I try to read Bernie Siegel's book. I try to think about Matthew's new house.

Matthew and I looked at houses together when I was out West skiing in early March. Matthew has been living in Breckenridge, Colorado, for about five years. He moved there after graduating from college with a music degree. He concentrated on developing a rock-and-jazz band for the first few years while selling time-shares in condos to pay the rent. We always knew that Matt's two older brothers would graduate from college. When Matthew made it down the aisle of the auditorium of Belmont University with "Colorado or bust" on the top of his mortarboard and the honor of being named to the dean's list his last semester, we had the biggest celebration in graduating Cheeks' history. Forget his father's Harvard degree. That was easy. Jim went into withdrawal when he finally had to leave school with the last of a few graduate degrees. He still teaches a class at Vanderbilt Law School no matter how busy his law practice. Academics were a constant challenge for Matthew, yet he had bravely conquered each hurdle. After four years in Colorado, he decided to try for his real-estate license and was now selling enough mountain houses and condominiums to support a surprisingly decent lifestyle. When Jim and I were first married, his parents gave us the down payment on our first house. This jump-start to savings and investments put us way ahead of the curve, and we had always been grateful. Since we could afford to pass on this favor to our children (and we felt they deserved it), we did the same. Our first down payment was for a house in Nashville for the oldest, Jamie. Next came Doctor Daniel's house in German Village in downtown Columbus, Ohio, at the beginning of his three-year medical residency. Now we would invest for our youngest son, Matthew, with a small wood-framed house at the base of his mountain.

I was excited about fluffing, buying a sofa and a few other furniture bits, and then making a hit at K-Mart for a small contribution of flatware, china, and some pots. Matthew and his girlfriend, Jessie, whom we adore, had been sharing digs with various friends for several years, and the early attic collection of furniture and accessories was stained and sagging and dismal.

They needed some new stuff for the new start. I was also thinking of every way I could of encouraging the relationship. Jim told me regularly to back off and mind my own business, but I'm a mom and this girl is terrific. We are all crazy about her. I know what I'm doing.

During the mornings and early afternoons of our three-day stay we sit in sofas, measure end tables and dressers, and break for lunches in Jessie and Matt's favorite hangouts, usually feeding friends of theirs as well. I love watching my son interact with all the people in this small town, the main street lined with painted Victorian houses. These grounded friends are now so much a part of his life. I rejoice in the place he has created for himself.

Each day by four, I retreat to the master bedroom of the new house for a restorative nap. Jim and I have been given the only bed. The room furnishings consist of a new king-size mattress and box springs and a crate of some sort to hold a rickety lamp. The first night, the kids sleep on the living room floor, buffered by a couple of blankets. The second day we buy an inflatable mattress. I feel no remorse. Why didn't they anticipate the need for an inflatable mattress? As soon as I close the door to the master bedroom, the silence folds over me and I move to an ever-increasing level of anxiety and fear. Each day, the coil in my stomach and the vice around my brain tighten with added tension. Sleeping pills help some at night, and so does the evening vino. I hide my feelings from the kids so they can keep their focus where I feel it should be, on the new house. Matthew cares deeply about his mom and calls often to hear how I am doing, but I don't want my fears taking over the space of this happy new setting. During the day I stay upbeat with shopping distractions, and behind closed doors I cry, thinking of the countdown to chemo.

On Sunday morning Jim's cell phone rings again. This time his hospital executive friend Jack and his wife, Barbara, are both on the phone, tag-teaming me, offering to set up a meeting with their oncologist. Barbara has just recovered from a second round of breast cancer. She points out, "I would have consulted anyone who could shed new light on my situation, and you don't even have to go out of town."

She is right. I give in, recognizing that I am lucky to have such a resource. Jack says to call him Monday morning at his office and gives me his private number. We head back to Nashville, leaving a happy twosome in the mountains waiting for furniture deliveries and already planning the deck with hot tub that they are going to have to pay for themselves.

On the plane back to Nashville, I think about a conversation from years ago with our oldest son, Jamie, when we were helping him move from college to the real world. Jim had used his pull to help him land a fabulous first job in New York City. Soon afterward, he was sitting next to me at dinner and said, "Mom, I feel guilty that I might have taken this job away from someone else who is more deserving." I answered, "I don't think you need to feel guilty about that. Opening doors is the way of the world. What you should feel guilty about is if you don't work extremely hard now that the door has been opened to do the best job you possibly can."

As I think about the door that has just been opened for me, I too feel guilty. On the day of discovery, I am in the office of the best oncologist at Vanderbilt, which is one of the leading cancer centers in the country. I am now offered a second opinion with no effort on my part from another top-notch oncologist. Is this fair?

Then I think of the commitment Jim and I have made to Nashville. Jim has been a valuable counselor to people who have contributed significantly to Nashville's business and political life. I have clocked untold hours raising money and developing programs for a wide range of nonprofits as a volunteer. Could I justify this as payback time for us? When this is over, I know I will need to figure out how I can give back to others with cancer who do not have access to the vast support team I enjoy. But for now, I will accept this opportunity to step through yet another opened door before I face my own chemo fight.

Back in Nashville, I meet with my priest, Ken. I had been going to his classes for years and was delighted to have the opportunity to visit with him one-on-one. I had built up a series of questions over years in his classes that I looked forward to "unpacking" (Ken's favorite word) with him one at a time. One of the best things our church offers is the plethora of stimulating, intellectually focused classes. As I struggled to put meaning and perspective on the road ahead, I relished the chance for private time with a spiritual companion whom I already knew and trusted. Ken and I had bonded soon after his arrival eight years ago to assume the position of Dean of Christ Church Cathedral. But hundreds of parishioners had bonded with Ken, and he was always so busy. I noticed other people meeting with him, one-on-one, but I didn't want to take up his time. Now I had an excuse to ask for personal attention. We had already built a relationship of mutual respect. I took comfort in this before my first meeting with him when I was a wreck, a complete wreck. I knew he would love me anyway. Now one of the first perks of cancer would be the opportunity to explore with Ken my new spiritual awakening.

When I pull into the parking lot of the cathedral the Monday after my return from Breckenridge and transition from the asphalt below my feet to the grey-stone facade in front of me, I am transported to England a few centuries back. Old is my thing. The church skin fits me like my boiled-wool bedroom slippers. I love the weathered stone exterior, the carved oak doors, the acanthus finials on each end of the mahogany pews. I love the center aisle lined with limestone columns, topped by carved capitals flaring out to form exotic geometric flowers.

Contests could be won over our stained-glass window collection. On Sundays, I sit where I can look up at the muted, golden tones of the window that came from the Tiffany glass factory in the 1920s.

The walls of the sanctuary, a luminous moss green, envelop me like a lush spring glade. And don't get me started on the music and Sunday morning flowers.

Thank God that before cancer I had found my church home. Writer and member of our congregation Robert Benson refers to our urban sanctuary as "an outpost of the promised land." The eclectic congregation is nurturing, the clergy intellectually engaging. This church community has become as important as my family and close friends, and having all three teams is strong ammunition for what lies ahead.

I had been part of Christ Church Cathedral in downtown Nashville for ten years, and as I reached into my soul to grasp any comforting life raft floating by, I realized that I had spent too much time floating on the surface of my spiritual life. At least I was comfortable with the congregation and clergy. At least I was familiar with the church rituals and routines, now that I really needed to talk to God. I felt as if I had the tools, but hadn't really taken the time to use them. Perhaps I hadn't needed to use them. Now that I was desperate, I was grateful to have a familiar spiritual home. I was grateful that I had taken Ken's prayer 101 class several years ago. Yet the suggested meditation prayers were an obstacle I had never conquered. Other people seemed to take to centering prayer or meditation, different variations on the same theme, with ease. The practice always eluded me. But after meditation, the next suggested practice was usually journaling. Other students in the class who were good at meditation spoke of not being able to journal. I wanted to raise my hand and say, "I can do that." Journaling came easily to me. I already knew that the place where I could tap into the richest part of me was through writing. I already knew that if I was conscious of God being with me, on my shoulder so to speak, as I concentrated on being completely honest and open and wrote with a positive spin, something magical would begin to happen.

At the beginning of my pilgrimage at Christ Church, I had attended a series of lectures on Thomas Merton, a pioneer monk whose writings were revered when I was a student at Manhattanville in the 1960s. After the first lecture, I searched through the church bookstore for Thomas Merton books and next to the *M*s on the shelf were books by Henri Nouwen. I had never heard of him, but as I was waiting to pay for a Merton biography, I picked up a copy of *Seeds of Hope*. I happened to open the book to page 28 where Nouwen writes:

> Writing is a process in which we discover what lives within us. The deepest satisfaction of writing is precisely that it opens up new spaces within us of which we were not aware before we started to write. To write is to embark on a journey whose final destination we do not know. Thus, writing requires a real act of trust. We have to say to ourselves, "I do not yet know what I carry in my heart, but I trust that it will emerge as I write." Writing is like giving away the loaves and the fishes one has, trusting that they will multiply in the giving.

Over the next few years I read everything I could find by Nouwen. I suppose others experience through meditation what Nouwen is talking about in this passage about writing, but my muse hovers somewhere between my fingers and the keyboard. I am not convinced that I will ever find my inner voice through silence, through contemplation. When I was in therapy, I discovered that if I wrote and wrote, if I let the words pour out on the page, they clarified my thinking on areas of my life from past to present. Journaling was where my core strength could grow. Journaling was a skill that I had honed for just this moment. Now the e-mails added an additional twist to the pen.

But meditation eludes me. At our meeting I tell Ken how difficult the practice of meditation is for me. He gives me an exercise: breathe in deeply and invite God into the space. With each exhaling breath, ask Him to take the anxiety away. I work on the exercise, thinking of the trauma of doctor and dentist visits at the beginning of the week, but feel nothing.

Wednesday morning, I go in to have the port inserted, a plastic disk about the size of a quarter that is put under the skin four inches below the collar bone with a small line that attaches directly into the jugular vein. Fortunately, strappy little sun or evening dresses are in my daughter-in-law's wardrobe, not mine. Jim is with me this time and I am prepared to be a wreck. I take a Valium a half hour before the surgery. When I lie down on the narrow hospital bed, I can't believe how calm I feel. Is it the pill? My blood pressure, which has been hovering at 160 over 90 or 95, is 138 over 78. How can this be after the anxiety I have sustained for so many weeks? Could the focus on deep breathing and being conscious of bringing God in and sending anxiety away finally be working? Could it really make such a difference? I can't believe how at ease I am as they finish the procedure and I awake from my twilight sleep. In the past, when I awoke in an operating room I would freak out, but this time I was in complete control. The sense of calm had lasted through the operation and was still with me. Could the meditation and deep breathing turn a nightmare into a bearable situation? Maybe it was the Valium that hadn't worn off.

Maybe it helped when I breathed God the Father in with the first breath; Jesus with the second; Sophia, the spirit and my feminine face of God with the third; and the Virgin Mother with the fourth. (I love a crowd and I needed all the help I could muster.) Maybe it was because I repeated the sequence over and over for the last two nights.

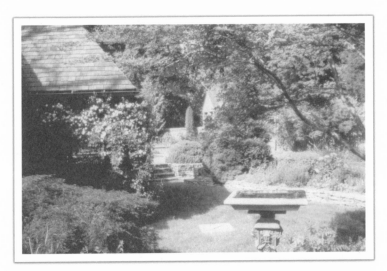

The birdbath and side garden outside our bedroom.

Whatever the reason, I had suddenly undergone a powerful transformation. I couldn't pinpoint the exact time when the change occurred. It had somehow snuck up on me. I was unaware of the change until I was lying on the bed before the port operation, and I noticed the anxiety was just gone. Gone. Would I be able to convey this phenomenon to the e-mail team? Oh, how I wanted to.

The night before chemo, I am walking in my garden at seven, waiting for Jim to come home with order-out dinner. The meals organized by my friend Carole won't start until after the first chemo session. The cat is beside me, rubbing against my leg. The fountain is spilling into the pool, and the robins are flying into the crepe myrtle over the birdbath in the crescent garden having evening conversation. The yellow 'Sunsprite' rose and the pale peach 'Peace' rose are fully opened, each petal of these early spring roses flawless. I cut a few to take with me in the morning. I use the rose scissors from the silver cup on the secretary in our bedroom and make the cuts just above a five-leaf connection, careful to avoid the lethal thorns.

I am ready. My arm is still sore from the lymph-biopsy surgery. Deal with that later. The new port feels like a foreign invader under my skin and is black and blue on either side, but I won't touch it.

With my amazing circle of friends, I know I will not be alone for the first chemo tomorrow. Dr. Greer's nurse practitioner, Ellen, has already been added to the contact list. We talked for forty-five minutes on Thursday afternoon, spending follow-up time that Dr. Greer would not have been able to give me. She, on the other hand, seemed to have all the time in the world to answer any leftover questions and to anticipate those I should have asked but didn't. She went over all of the meds I needed before starting chemo. So confusing. She told me to take a Compazine tonight for nausea and another in the morning. She told me to take an Ambien and a Benadryl for sleeping. She told me to take half a tranquilizer in the morning, which I didn't need, and half a pain pill, which I did. I tried to remember if I had ever taken more than two pills together, other than vitamins, in my life.

I will sleep again tonight with the meds Ellen recommends. I will leave tomorrow fortified with the meds Ellen recommends. I will be free of most surprises because Ellen has gone carefully over the drill: nausea ifs, bathroom ifs, insomnia ifs. The role played by a competent nurse practitioner has eased the doctor's load and enhanced support for the patient. I thank whoever is responsible for adding this new position to the health-support team. I will come back this evening to my garden and have more roses and peonies opening, another at its peak, another bird to listen to, my tabby cat to keep me company.

Chemo One

*T*he next morning I arrive at the Vanderbilt Cancer Center at 7:30, wait until 8:00 to be put in a room, have the blood extracted at 8:15 and sent to the lab, and then wait for the results to be sent to Dr. Greer's office to confirm that my blood counts are strong enough to go ahead with the procedure and to write the prescription for the drug cocktail called CHOP+R: C for Cytoxan, H for Adriamycin or doxorubicin (don't ask me why—neither starts with an H), O for Oncovin or vincristine, P for prednisone, given orally at the beginning of the session, and R for Rituxan, which I am told will take the last two hours to administer. Everything is carefully planned, carefully timed.

Then we wait again for the chemo cocktail to be mixed and sent back down to me, sitting patiently in the Barcalounger. The meds arrive at ten o'clock, three and a half hours after I was told to be there. Hospital hours. I must be thankful they are cautious. I must also be thankful that I seem not to have an issue with low blood counts. Many patients choose to have blood work done the day before a procedure to determine if they can proceed or if they need to wait and have a blood transfusion to boost the numbers in their white blood-cell count. When other leukemia patients ask me about my white blood count, I don't know the numbers, as it has never been an issue.

Believe it or not, the nurse starts off my chemo session by giving me two extra-strength Tylenol and Benadryl and then the steroid pill prednisone for pain and nausea before starting the bags of three liquid drugs and one more in a large hypodermic needle, which they "push" in. The nasty drugs drip slowly into my body for the rest of the day. The bags of liquid poison slide down a plastic tube, slowly entering my jugular vein, accessed directly by way of the new port. I wait to feel the burn, the nausea, something. I am there until four-thirty.

I am back in the film, scene 2. The director is behind my left shoulder and will soon say, "Cut." I will take the fake needle out of my chest, where there will be no mark, and will go back to my garden and overprogrammed, volunteer marathon life.

I have friends lined up who want to go with me to chemo. Just as Carole organizes meals, Connie has organized an amazing team divided into three shifts to sit with me and distract me from the drip. Jim and the e-mail queen, Linda, are there for the beginning of the session. As legal advisor to boards of directors of companies in Nashville and beyond, Jim's schedule remains hectic. I understand that he cannot be there to hold my hand for the duration of each session. I know being the nurturer at bedside is not his strong suit anyway. The team of friends is better and crucial for my many trips to the doctors and treatments. I feel too woozy to read or needle-point, and mostly we visit or I doze and the time passes surprisingly quickly. I think about what I will do when all of this is over. I will take time out. I will live in the moment. I will walk every day as I begin to redefine "Patient Siggy." I already sense I will not go back to my old routine. I breathe deeply and open a space at the bottom of my diaphragm, and watch the word "peace" written in pale pink, the color of the peony, float in an arch above my head.

Last night I reread one of Ken's lessons about the Greek word for inner peace, *apathia*. Ken had reminded me about the word at our meeting. Apathia is the state of feeling everything, but not allowing it to control us. We remain free. During the onset of pain, anguish, and anxiety, we have the opportunity to reach down and find inner strength, to feel something stirring in us, just out of sight, to help us through the difficult time. When we are feeling better, we forget to concentrate enough to feel this inner strength. Ken has told the Christ Church congregation that apathia is the most valued virtue of the Desert Fathers, the first monks in the early church who went to the desert to imitate the life of Christ, but apathia is also the hardest virtue to understand. Once a person experiences this virtue, he or she will never forget it. I close my eyes and try to think about the free part of me that doesn't need to be focused on the needles, on the flu-like aches, on the headache beginning just above my eyes.

As I receive chemo, the three roses from my garden sit beside me in a small vase. How can there be so many color variations within the subtle palate of blush pinks and yellows? The last drug, Rituxan, is the most powerful, and indeed, takes two hours to slowly drip from the plastic sack hung from a metal stand, down the plastic tube, through the port, and into my veins. The nurse, Michele, starts the drug slowly. Each half hour, a beeper goes off and she returns to ratchet up the dosage, monitoring how well I tolerate each increase. The last half hour, the dosage is so strong that I imagine having to take a wheelchair to get to the car. The last of the liquid is inside me, and I think about bad cells hovering under the swollen area under my arm being zapped by my army of liquid soldiers. I rest for fifteen minutes while they flush the port with a saline solution, and surprisingly, I revive. I am able to walk unassisted. I give the three roses to Michele on the way out. After a few more steps, I decide that I am strong enough to visit Bill. Connie and I walk over to the Stallworth wing of the hospital and peek in on Nicky's husband, who is in the hospital for a week of testing. I make it down the long corridor, and we visit for five minutes. I think of the years and years that Bill has had to deal with hospital procedures, and yet he greets me with a cheerful face and an "I'm fine, m'dear. How are you?"

Connie then drives me home and I ask her to make one more detour a few blocks from the hospital to stop in front of a small, brick house with a wrought-iron fence on Fairfax Avenue. I have passed the five-foot-tall poppies and watched them open and mature on my various visits to the hospital. They are in the back of my mind during the treatment as I plan my heist. I know that the poppy pods will be forming. I get out of the car and reach over the fence and pull off about twelve pods. It's OK, I think. My garden needs more poppies.

I steal garden seeds. I promise I don't steal anything else, but seeds I steal in abundance. Poppy pods are easy to snag, and each small pod contains hundreds of seeds. Heck, I've even stolen poppy seeds from Monet's garden in Giverny—tricky but doable. I've stolen grape hyacinth seeds from the neighbor's mailbox. Cleome is another good seed to steal, but I have plenty. You can come steal that one from me. I am relentless in my search for poppy seeds to add to my garden. Seeds are always in abundance, and so many are left behind to be trampled and abandoned. I say good for me and other gardeners to resurrect a few more seeds from oblivion, put them in a labeled envelope, save them, and then spread them across February snow and watch them mysteriously transform in early spring to tiny, green leaves pushing out of the black earth, helping spread nature's abundance from one garden to another. You must bend over and thin the numerous poppy sprouts so they have space to recreate their majestic five-foot stems and four-inch blossoms before they, too, gently bend over like miniature swans and become another egg-shaped seed pod. I will be here—I will *absolutely* be here—next May to pick those recycled pods and put them in another envelope and share. Peonies take years to establish and hate to be moved or divided, but the poppy is portable and easy to plant. There are plenty for all of us. They will never be missed. There are hundreds more.

Then I am home. I put on my coziest pink-knit pajamas. I contemplate the poppy seeds I have just snatched and sleep. I sleep for twelve hours. The next day I spend in bed, slightly nauseated, but by the next I revive enough for another e-mail update.

With the e-mail team I want to plant the essence, hit the highlights: the end of trips, the dentist visit, the last visit with Dr. Greer, Ken's breathing exercises and their amazing effects, and my upcoming haircut.

UPDATE FROM PATIENT SIGGY
MAY 16, 2005
DEAR FRIENDS,

AFTER THE RETURN FROM A WONDERFUL WEEKEND IN COLORADO AND SEEING OUR YOUNGEST SO HAPPY WITH A NEW HOUSE AND A REAL JOB, HITTING REALITY WAS HARD. I KNEW IT WAS TIME TO FACE THE MUSIC: THE TRIP TO FLORIDA OVER—CHECK; THE TRIP TO NYC OVER—CHECK; THE OUTRAGEOUSLY EXPENSIVE SHOES CHARGED—CHECK. THERE WAS A CARTOON IN *The New Yorker* LAST WEEK WITH A WOMAN LOOKING INTO A SHOE-STORE WINDOW WITH THE TAG LINE, "EVERY JOURNEY SHOULD START WITH AN EXPENSIVE PAIR OF NEW SHOES." I WAS HOME FOR THE BEGINNING OF MY JOURNEY, CHEMO STARTING ON FRIDAY.

I WAS TOO PREOCCUPIED AND TIRED TO WRITE THE FIRST WEEK AFTER RETURNING FROM COLORADO. I HAD TESTS EVERY DAY AND THE MID-WEEK MEETING WITH DR. GREER LEFT ME FILLED WITH ANXIETY.

I USED TO THINK THAT VANDERBILT HOSPITAL WAS A MYSTERIOUS MASS OF BRICK THAT HAD NOTHING TO DO WITH ME. ON LAST MONDAY, I WALKED INTO THE RADIOLOGY DEPARTMENT ON THE FIRST FLOOR, RIGHT BEHIND THE MAIN LOBBY OF THE HOSPITAL, FAMILIAR WITH THE DRILL. I HAD BEEN THERE SEVERAL TIMES. YOU NAME THE TEST. I BET I'VE HAD IT.

I KNOW WHERE TO PARK FOR THE CLINIC, ROY'S OFFICE, DR. GREER'S OFFICE, AND VARIOUS LABS. I KNOW WHAT TO DO IF IT'S

TOO EARLY FOR THE GUY TO BE AT THE BOOTH TO STAMP THE PARKING TICKET. I KNOW THAT THE HENRY JOYCE CANCER CENTER IS UNDER THE CLINIC WITH A CROSSWALK ON THE SECOND FLOOR OF THE PARKING GARAGE ACROSS THE STREET. I KNOW THE BREAST CANCER CENTER IS ACROSS 21ST AVENUE IN ANOTHER BUNCH OF BRICK BUILDINGS CALLED THE VILLAGE OF VANDERBILT.

I LOST IT THE WEEK BEFORE BRECKENRIDGE WHEN I HAD A TEST IN THE RADIOLOGY LAB AND THEY GAVE ME TOO MANY CHOICES FOR THE WAY I COULD HAVE A NEEDLE. I LOST IT ON MONDAY WHEN I WENT TO THE DENTIST FOR TEETH CLEANING (ROUTINE BEFORE CHEMO) AND HAD TO HAVE A CROWN. MY BLOOD PRESSURE WAS SKY-HIGH.

I KNEW I WOULD BE GOING TO DR. GREER FOR THE FINAL MEDICAL PLAN ON WEDNESDAY, BUT I NEEDED A SPIRITUAL PLAN AS WELL. I MET WITH KEN, DEAN OF CHRIST CHURCH CATHEDRAL AND MY SPIRITUAL MENTOR, ON TUESDAY AFTERNOON. HE LISTENED TO A LONG LIST OF ANXIETY-RIDDEN CONCERNS. HE REMINDED ME OF THE CLASSES I HAD TAKEN TO LEARN ABOUT MEDITATION. I HADN'T GOTTEN IT. I COULD JOURNAL, BUT MEDITATE? HE REMINDED ME TO ENTER INTO A PLACE OF QUIET AND STILLNESS. NOT MY STRONG POINT. BREATHE DEEPLY. ASK GOD TO COME IN. THEN GIVE GOD THE ANXIETY. FILL THE SPACE WITH PEACE. HE HUGGED ME AND TOLD ME THAT HE WOULD BE WITH ME EVERY STEP OF THE WAY.

I WENT HOME THAT NIGHT AND TRIED TO THINK ABOUT THE BREATHING AND STILLNESS, BUT I COULDN'T FIND THE SPACE. I WOKE AT ABOUT THREE. I TRIED THE BREATHING AND THE PRAYERS. IT WASN'T WORKING. I WOKE AT FOUR. I BREATHED DEEPLY INTO MY DIAPHRAGM, OVER AND OVER. I TRIED THINKING ABOUT GOD FILLING THE SPACE AND TAKING AWAY MY ANXIETY. THIS WASN'T WORKING. AT SIX I TRIED AGAIN. AT LEAST THE DEEP BREATHING WAS BETTER THAN WHAT I WOULD HAVE BEEN THINKING ABOUT INSTEAD.

I WENT TO HAVE THE PORT PUT IN WEDNESDAY MORNING AT SEVEN-THIRTY. FUNNY, I FELT CALM, RELAXED. THEY TOOK MY BLOOD PRESSURE. IT HAD GONE DOWN TWENTY POINTS. I FELT POWERFUL. THEY PUT ME IN A TWILIGHT SLEEP FOR THE PROCE-DURE. AS THEY WERE FINISHING UP I AWOKE AND SPOKE CALMLY TO THE DOCTORS. I KNEW EVERYTHING WOULD BE FINE.

I FELT THE SAME PEACE THE DAY OF THE CHEMO. ROY CAME BY AND I BRAGGED ABOUT MY BLOOD PRESSURE AND TOLD HIM ABOUT THE MEDITATION. HE TOLD ME THAT BREATHING DEEPLY INTO THE

DIAPHRAGM HAS BEEN PROVEN TO CAUSE A CHEMICAL REACTION. SCIENCE OR MIRACLE? YOUR PICK. THE TREATMENT COULD HAVE LASTED EIGHT HOURS, BUT AS I HAD NO ADVERSE EFFECTS FROM THE DRUGS, ALL PROCEEDED IN AN EFFICIENT MANNER AND I WAS FINISHED IN SIX. ONLY THE LAST FORTY MINUTES WERE UNPLEASANT. WHEN THEY WERE FINISHED, I WAS ABLE TO RALLY, WALK OUT, AND GO HOME TO MY LITTLE BED. THE NEXT DAY HAD A FEW ROUGH SPOTS, BUT I AM DOING GREAT. I CAN'T BELIEVE THAT THE LUMPS UNDER MY ARMS ARE ALMOST GONE. I WILL LICK THIS. I AM SURE.

TOMORROW I AM GOING TO HAVE MY HAIR CUT REALLY SHORT. I HAVE ALWAYS WONDERED WHAT THAT WOULD LOOK LIKE AND I WOULD NEVER HAVE HAD THE NERVE TO GIVE IT A TRY. I'M TURNING MY HAIR SITUATION INTO AN OPPORTUNITY. BLOND WIGS HAVE ALSO BEEN SUGGESTED AND THEY ARE DEFINITELY UNDER CONSIDERATION. I DO HAVE A NIFTY MAGENTA ONE THAT I BOUGHT IN SOHO A FEW YEARS AGO.

I AM TIRED BUT PUMPED. AND, YOU STILL HAVE TO BE NICE TO ME FOR A WHILE. KEEP PRAYERS COMING.

HUGS, SIGOURNEY

I wish I could better explain the sudden change from anxiety to calm. I know it is not just a coincidence that after a month of anxiety, I am able to handle the port operation and the beginning of chemo with such a peaceful demeanor. I certainly had felt no bolt of lightening, no connection with a greater power. Yet when I was lying on the table before the port surgery, the anxiety that had been a steady companion was no longer there. The cavity of tension was replaced by an aura of peace and well-being. Was it the deep breathing? I think so. Was it all the people who were praying for me? I think so. Is there a logical explanation or was God just staying invisible?

One friend is anything but invisible. The first response in my e-mail inbox had been from Carole, who has used my contact list to create "Sigourney's Meals on Wheels." She writes:

DEAR ALL,

OF COURSE I LOVE TO RUN THINGS SO I HAVE BECOME THE MEAL DEPOT COORDINATOR—I KNOW MOST OF YOU KNOW THIS—BUT JUST A BIT MORE INFORMATION—SIGOURNEY GOES IN TOMORROW FOR EIGHT HOURS OF CHEMOTHERAPY. PUTTING IN THE PORT YESTERDAY WAS NOT TOO BAD—SHE WAS TIRED BUT FELT PRETTY WELL LAST NIGHT. WE HAVE FRIENDS WITH HER ALL DAY TOMORROW FOR THE EIGHT HOURS—READERS, KNITTERS, NEEDLEWORKERS, LISTENERS, ETC . . . SO THAT IS COVERED. WE ARE STARTING OUR PROCESS OF MEALS ON MONDAY—WE WILL HAVE A MON/THURS/SAT ROTATION—AND WE WILL PUT A LARGE COOLER ON HER BACK PORCH SO THAT WE CAN SIMPLY DROP OFF OUR MEALS AND NOT BOTHER SLEEP, ETC. PLEASE, PLEASE PUT DIRECTIONS ON HOW TO PREPARE—HEATING, ETC . . . AND PUT YOUR NAME ON IT SO SHE WILL KNOW WHO BROUGHT WHAT—I WILL KEEP A COPY OF IT TOO FOR HER. IF YOU ARE AN OUT-OF-TOWN FRIEND, I CAN EASILY GIVE YOU NUMBERS (OR CALL FOR YOU) OF CATERERS ETC . . . AND A LOT OF TIME WE SIMPLY ORDER FROM OUR COUNTRY CLUB AND JIM OR JAMIE CAN PICK UP. SHE LOVES YOU ALL FOR THIS—AND IT IS A CHANCE FOR ALL OF US TO CONTRIBUTE TO A DEAR, DEAR FRIEND. SHE LOVES HEARING FROM YOU TOO—BUT NOTES AND CARDS ARE PROBABLY BETTER THAN PHONE CALLS TO RETURN . . . WHAT AM I FORGETTING??? HERE ARE THE DATES THROUGH JUNE— E-MAIL ME BACK WHEN YOU MIGHT BE ABLE TO FILL IN—SINCE THERE ARE BOUND TO BE DUPLICATIONS, I WILL E-MAIL YOU BACK TO CONFIRM THE DATE . . . AND TELL THOSE WHO DIDN'T . . . AND THANKS SO MUCH.

CAROLE

A list of dates follows in a single column making it easy for people to sign up. What a friend, keeping up with all of this and making my meal life stress-free for the duration of my chemo treatments through the end of July. Anne delivers a big cooler that lives on the back porch to be opened every other day with another sumptuous meal. Does the support of loving friends add to my peace of mind? I think so.

True Confession

I don't know why I say I was in chemo for six hours in the e-mail. I was there for nine. Maybe it is part of a denial syndrome. Maybe I was just counting the actual time it took to administer the drugs. Maybe it is that adjusting to hospital time is endless, so you stop paying attention.

What I also spare the e-mail team are the details of how totally out of control I was at the dentist, the Monday before I had chemo. The hygienist made me jump when she touched an upper, back molar, and I knew I was in trouble. I had broken off one of the four corners of a molar a few months back and I put it on the list of things I usually ignore, and besides, I felt no pain when I chewed on the other side. My dentist, Gary, came in to reprobe and confirmed that I would need a crown. When he reached for the Novocain shot, my body went rigid. I started to shake, to vibrate like the massage recliner on display at the Brookstone store. Tears started to flow. I recognized the strange response my body exhibits under extreme distress. I remember that strange sensation from when I was giving birth to Jamie, during the pre-examination for my hysterectomy, and after a bad car accident three years ago. I shook all over, like a vibrator, unable to stop. Now it took the last of my energy to say to Gary, "Do . . . do you ha . . . have so . . . some of that la . . . laughing ga . . . gas?" I remembered my last root canal had been almost heaven with the use of this amazing drug. Now it barely made a dent. I felt an unpleasant, metallic taste in my mouth. I asked the nurse if I could hold her hand. I was nowhere near the la-la land I remembered from the root canal, but time did pass more quickly as I held on for dear life. Gary opened yet another door. A real crown, which usually takes ten days to make, would be ready on Thursday morning before Friday's chemo.

When I left the dentist, I noticed a message on my cell phone from Anne. I called back to see if she was still home and told her I was coming right over. I couldn't face going home to an empty house after the tooth trauma. I didn't usually have trauma attacks. I broke down again on her front door step. After calming down, I told her about the Monday 8:00 AM call to our friend Jack who had offered to call his hospital for a second opinion, and the 8:15 response from his doctor for a 1:30 afternoon appointment today. I had to pull myself back together and go.

She rearranged her day and took me to the appointment. We increased the forces by picking up Anne Taylor on the way. (I want to step out of the story at this point and tell you, if you are sick and have a friend who wants to help, say thank you and let her. You will both receive a gift.) When the nurse called me into the office, I gathered all my reports, asked both ladies to come with me, and said, "They are my committee." They both had pads and pens. The doctor agreed with most of the reports. He was not convinced that Richter's was the correct diagnosis. He suggested that the transformation to a larger-cell lymphoma could have possibly been caused by the infectious bug bites. The presence of a larger cancer was definitely correct, and he concurred with the CHOP+R treatment. He did, however, feel that it was important to consider a PET scan before the chemo. This test magnifies the places in the body where cancer exists. After the first four treatments, I could have another PET scan and determine the exact effectiveness of the chemo. We left with two detailed sets of notes, grateful for the doctor's time and advice.

What I also didn't tell the e-mail team was how I freaked out when I had a message on the answering machine confirming my port operation for Wednesday when I had been told it would be on Thursday, the day before the chemo. Did that mean the chemo was Thursday? The message was on the answering machine: "To confirm this appointment press one, to reschedule press two." I couldn't press anything listening to the answering machine. Would they cancel the appointment because I wasn't there to press one? I called. No, the chemo was on Friday. They guessed the port was scheduled for Wednesday because there were no scheduled times on Thursday. The conflict you feel when a dreaded event that you are finally facing is not going to take place when you thought it was is wrenching. Juggling crucial times for treatments and hearing about it on a recording only add to mounting anxiety. It takes weeks to assume the right mindset for an operation. You want everything on schedule, under control, fine-tuned, in perfect balance before you walk into the hospital to be cut open.

I also didn't tell the e-mail team about the appointment with Dr. Greer after the port operation on Wednesday to confirm all our options before having chemo on Friday. After conferring with colleagues at M.D. Anderson and Sloan Kettering, Dr. Greer concluded that even though my symptoms were less severe than most with my diagnosis, all the pathology reports confirmed I did have Richter's syndrome, and he recommended the most aggressive chemo treatment, CHOP+R. I leaned forward at the end of my checklist of questions, "What about considering a PET scan as a baseline before chemo?" He pushed his wheeled chair closer to the computer screen and looked at my data. "I think we will schedule a PET scan for tomorrow."

As it turns out, we were lucky to have the port out of the way on Wednesday and have Thursday free for the PET, a two-hour procedure. No matter how good the doctors—and I had the best—they see so many patients each day. You have to be your own advocate. Maybe the PET scan is not essential, but it is going to be an important addition to my peace of mind.

Recovery from Chemo One

*M*y life has changed again, another turn, another rethinking of our routine. A month ago, we told Jamie and Lisa we would take grandson Jack to Ponte Vedra for the weekend so they could take a much-deserved trip. Lisa's mom has agreed to keep baby Baker. After the first chemo, I know a weekend away with a two-year-old isn't the best choice for recuperation. Jim suggests we stay at our house in Nashville and have Jack here. Jim says he'll take care of him. Jim is great for short periods, but I am not confident about his staying power over a weekend, and I am in no condition to pick up the slack. I can't even lift Jack with my sore chest and arm from the various surgeries. Lisa's mother, the best grandmother ever, steps in and agrees to keep both grandchildren. I will find that seeing less of my grandchildren with my fatigue and the risks of catching an infection from their childhood ailments is another downside of chemo. A stronger susceptibility to infection is another symptom of CLL.

When I feel nausea the first few nights, I wake up, go to the kitchen, and suck on a piece of pickled ginger. That helps. I take another Ambien sleeping pill. I am restless, but relaxed. The steroids I have to take for five days constantly interrupt sleep. I take an extra-strength Tylenol for a persistent headache, but aside from these minor issues, I am surprisingly symptom free. I can't take anything with aspirin as I am on a mild dose of Coumadin because of the foreign object, the port, inside my chest.

I am lucky to be going through chemo in 2005 when so many new drugs prevent the severe nausea of earlier years. The worst for me is the feeling of being bone tired. It's a debilitating tired that by early afternoon leaves me without energy to do anything more than get in bed and sleep again for a few hours, only to wake up with little energy for the rest of the day. How do people go back to work while undergoing this strong of a chemo treatment? I know many have no choice.

I am lucky to be under the care of Dr. Roy and lucky he was able to make an instantaneous connection with Dr. Greer. Looking back, what Dr. Greer executes to perfection is the ability to read a patient's response and sensitivity to information. He knows what should be done, but he gives a range of possible ways to proceed. For the newly indoctrinated into illness, the options and choices are as daunting as the vocabulary, too much information coming too fast to absorb. He lets you in on the selection of possibilities. He gives you time to assimilate the information and the consequences of the chosen action. He quietly suggests, "Let's schedule the procedure for a week from now just in case," giving you time to sit with the facts and come at your own pace to his recommendation. Then, the procedure is in the system, ready for you to just show up.

My time between treatments passes quietly. Every day someone leaves another surprise at my door, a note, flowers, even six bottles of Evian. After chemo, my taste for wine has taken a vacation.

A construction-paper picture made with colored pens is a get-well greeting from young boys, Cheek cousins who live next door to Jamie and Lisa, along with a plate of oatmeal and cherry chocolate cookies from their mom. Jim's ninety-two-year-old cousin takes the time to come over for a visit and share books about cancer and recipes, driving by herself, walking up the three front, railless steps by herself. I am writing hundreds of thank-you notes and don't make a dent as the gifts keep coming.

Linda brings me pomegranate juice, one of the best antioxidants. Several glasses diluted with water has replaced my mid-morning and early-afternoon Diet Dr Pepper. The drugs have killed my taste for wine and coffee. I start each morning with green tea and take the pomegranate juice to a dinner with friends at Anne and John's house. In a wine glass, it looks just like merlot.

I have had several offers of marijuana, but I don't think so. Thank God nausea is no longer the worst part. I know from various conversations with other cancer patients that some people still suffer from this malady, but the new meds have made nausea a minor issue for me. I would be skeptical about the marijuana anyway because I hallucinated for three days after some strong stuff I tried in the early '70s. With my one stab at marijuana, I sunk into a paranoid state thinking the world was out to get me and everyone I encountered was conspiring behind my back. My children don't believe me when I say this happened after one joint, but how could I make that up? It must have been powerful stuff. I'm not taking any chances of going there again, even though I received a manila envelope from anonymous "Christ Church Angels" with a dried marijuana plant and paper to roll a joint. I'll stick with meditation attempts and sleeping pills. Dr. Roy has warned me to avoid unnecessary fatigue at all cost.

Carole's food brigade comes religiously three times a week with meals scheduled through July, and people are lined up for slots. I can't believe it. One of the perks of Southern living, I am convinced.

I drag myself to the computer in the afternoon to check the messages that keep me going.

After my usual bridge on Tuesday, I take that one proactive step for hair. My hair texture is fine—not meaning OK—meaning limp.

My hair wants to flop down in the front of my eyes even if I've been to the hairdresser. I want to go back a few hours later and say, "See. The carefully combed-back front doesn't last, even with armor hair spray." I have always needed to be able to slip it behind an ear and forget about the hairdresser. Shoulder length was as short as I dare go. But now that I will lose it anyway, I figure I might as well be daring and go all out and cut, cut, cut. Besides, short hair falling out will be less traumatic. I go to the hair house once or twice a year for some fancy do, and so David can fuss about my slightly uneven trim self-executed every six weeks or so, using a hand mirror and a fabulous pair of scissors from my top dressing-room drawer that I use only for hair. I have some standards.

David loves being in charge of my shearing. The bridge group comes with me, standing in a semicircle and looking on with approval and applause.

A Spiritual High

I meet with Ken again on Wednesday. I tell him that after the calm following deep breathing, I am zoned in to each moment. I tell him about waking from the port surgery, talking to the doctors in a relaxed state, only curious about the details of what was happening. And for the first time in a hospital, I feel totally focused with no anxiety, no panic. Who is this person? I tell him I feel a new, powerful connection with God. I feel He is beside me throughout the day. I no longer have anything to fear. It is wondrous and peaceful at the same time. In the car, I keep the radio off and let my thoughts and amazing sense of calm roll over me. Ken replies, "Enjoy it while you can, for it will not last." I sense he is right, but for the moment I will bask in the peace. Ken suggests an exercise for the week: "Find a place of deep silence and quiet. Feel what it is like to be touched by the heart of God and hold yourself in that place, enjoy the feeling."

I tell Ken about the PET scan I had right before the first chemo, and about going alone and the drawing of more blood, the mixing with more radioactive stuff that is returned to my system to highlight all the places the aggressive cancer has spread in order to compare the results in three months, and again in six months. I tell him I am OK under the machines now. I no longer want to anesthetize my brain or be distracted. I want to face the news head-on, between the eyes, whatever the challenges. We discuss dealing with crisis, choosing to stay frozen with fear or to embrace the challenge and grow. I affirm, "I lived in the first mode for the first month. Plan B is better."

I love the mellow place that I have settled into as anxiety gives way to the inner peace I have found through a heightened appreciation and awareness of ordinary things. I no longer feel like a stand-in actor in a play whose part will soon end. I have assumed the permanent role. I have embraced the role. The part is who I am, who I was meant to be. I don't want to miss a scene, even if traumatic events have been saved for a big finish.

Dinner with Friends

Friday night, Jim and I go to a gathering of ten friends for dinner. The guys even make a fuss over my snappy, short haircut. "I love it. I hope you leave it that way," John says.

We all go out on the terrace of Anne and John's new house to a canopy pavilion with wicker armchairs at the end of the pool. The spring night temperature is ideal for alfresco dining. The stars, bright in the sky, complete the setting. The gravity of my disease seems to intensify the special bond we have shared over thirty plus years. When our host has filled orders for wine choices, we raise a glass to celebrate extraordinary friendships. Every person seems aware of the poignancy of our first gathering since my diagnosis, and a sacred quality hovers in the silence as we sip.

I remember the loss of the wife of one of our closest friends five years ago to a devastating disease. I received condolence letters, and she wasn't even a relative. Several months later, I was sitting next to a friend at a meeting, and she turned to me and told me she had been thinking of me and was sorry for my loss. She has a big family in Nashville, and I said, "Thank you so much for those kind words, but surely at our age we all experience something similar." She replied, "Not really. I don't know of anyone with the same friendships that your close friends share." She was right. Our close friends are an extraordinary group of achievement-oriented individuals with an uncanny bond. The mutual admiration, respect, and love we share is a gift all of us treasure.

When we sit for dinner, instead of discussing the score of the football game, a recent book, or how good a job the mayor is doing, I move the conversation to a deeper level. I share my extraordinary experience of new inner peace that has taken up residence in my being since last week and my deep-breathing meditation. I tell my end of the table I feel the peace of thousands of prayers: the prayers from the people at our church, the prayers passed on to other people with other prayer lists at other churches, even the prayers in other cities where my e-mails spread the word about my first treatment. Somehow, writing down my experience has added clarity to my journey and given me the words and courage to describe the power I feel surrounding me. Never would I have plucked at deep crevices in my heart in mixed company in the past. The next morning I call to thank our hostess, and she tells me her husband said the conversation at our end of the table was remarkable, like nothing in his memory.

A week after chemo I write another update, happy to be able to respond to so many with a click of the Send command. The efficiency of this high-tech communication is a joy; the contact list is up to eighty people.

UPDATE FROM PATIENT SIGGY
SATURDAY, MAY 21, 2005
DEAR FRIENDS,
EVERY DAY I COME HOME TO ANOTHER BEAUTIFUL NOTE FROM ANOTHER FRIEND WHO IS A WRITER AND MAYBE DOESN'T KNOW IT. HAND-PICKED FLOWERS FROM SOMEONE'S GARDEN ARE WEDGED BEHIND THE FRONT GLASS DOOR. ANOTHER FLORIST IS RINGING THE BACK DOORBELL. SOMEONE FROM CAROLE'S FOOD BRIGADE HAS LEFT A DELICIOUS DINNER. MY BIGGEST SMILE CAME FROM JANE'S SIMPLE SIX BOTTLES OF EVIAN, IN A BROWN BOX, FLUFFED WITH BLUE TISSUE AND A NOTE EXPLAINING THAT SHE UNDERSTOOD THAT THIS WAS MY CURRENT BEVERAGE OF CHOICE.

I TRIED TO TELL CAROLE THAT I DIDN'T REALLY NEED THE
DINNERS, BUT SHE TOLD ME TO SHUT UP AND ENJOY, AND BESIDES,
PEOPLE WANTED TO DO SOMETHING.

PEOPLE DON'T WANT TO BOTHER ME, BUT I WANT TO BE
BOTHERED. I LIKE ALL OF THE ATTENTION AND I AM GETTING
STRONGER. I'M WALKING EVERY DAY AND SEEKING COMPANIONSHIP.
I DID THREE MILES YESTERDAY WITH EUGENIA. I TALK TO OR SEE
NICKY AND CONNIE EVERY DAY. MARY JANE, CAROLE H., AND
LINDA CAME OVER THE DAY BEFORE YESTERDAY AND WE HUNG OUT
IN THE GARDEN FROM 4 TO 5:15. WHY DO I HAVE TO BE SICK TO
ENJOY A PERFECT SPRING DAY WITH THE PEONIES AND ROSES
STRETCHING OUT TO TAKE A BOW?

THE DAY BEFORE THAT, ON TUESDAY, MY BRIDGE GROUP AND
MARCELLA MET OVER AT TRUMPS. THEY STOOD BEHIND DAVID IN A
SEMICIRCLE, AS MY HAIR WAS LOPPED OFF SHORTER THAN NICKY'S.
DAVID SAID, "I'VE ALWAYS WANTED TO TRY THIS." HE WAS HAVING A
BETTER TIME THAN WE WERE. SOME OF THE OTHER GUYS AT TRUMPS
WERE CHECKING OUT THE COMMOTION. JAMES BROUGHT HIS HANDS
TO HIS EARS IN AN UPWARD MOTION AND SAID, "IT LIFTS YOUR FACE
UP ON THE SIDES." COULD THIS BE A CHEAP FACE-LIFT? I WAS SO
TIRED THAT AFTERNOON, THEN I STARTED FEELING PERKY AND LOVED
THE FUSS. I'M GOING TO MISS THE ATTENTION WHEN THE CANCER
DISAPPEARS AND I TURN BACK INTO A PUMPKIN.

YESTERDAY, DAVID REFLUFFED MY HAIR, AND LAST NIGHT, PERKY
ME WENT OUT TO DINNER FOR THE FIRST TIME WITH A FEW FRIENDS.
WE RAISED OUR GLASSES TO TOAST THIRTY-PLUS EXTRAORDINARY YEARS
OF FRIENDSHIP. MORE THAN ANYTHING, WE TREASURE OUR WIDE GROUP
OF FRIENDS WHO MUTUALLY LOVE AND RESPECT EACH OTHER. I AM
BLESSED TO FEEL UP TO THIS OCCASION, THAT HAS SOMEHOW TAKEN ON
A HEIGHTENED ENJOYMENT, A DEEPER CELEBRATION, AS MY ILLNESS
REMINDS US ALL OF UNIQUE BLESSINGS.

LAST WEEK I MET AGAIN WITH KEN FOR OUR WEEKLY VISIT. IF
SPIRITUALITY MAKES YOU WANT TO SHIVER INSTEAD OF SETTLING IN,
YOU CAN DELETE THIS PART.

I SPOKE TO KEN ABOUT THE SENSE OF PEACE THAT HAS SETTLED
INTO MY BEING AND SEEMS TO HAVE TAKEN UP RESIDENCE SINCE
LAST WEEK'S AMATEUR ATTEMPT AT DEEP-BREATHING MEDITATION.
THE CHEMICAL REACTION FROM DEEP BREATHING, UPON FURTHER
INQUIRY, RELEASES THE SAME ENDORPHINS THAT OCCUR WITH
VIGOROUS EXERCISE.

I asked Ken how I could continue to feel this peace and calm. I can't believe this could happen to someone so filled with anxiety and fear. For the month after the diagnosis, I went from denial to distraction: pickling my brain with bottles of white wine, popping pain pills and sleeping pills, preferably together, tuning out to multiple movie marathons. I asked him to explain the about-face.

Ken answered, "Thousands of people are praying for you." "What?" I said. "Think about your e-mails going out and the number of people who then send it on to someone else." I thought of our church and friends from other churches, large churches, who said that they had put me on a prayer list. I started seeing lists of people growing.

Ken said, "You are surrounded by people praying for you." He made a gesture of a huge embrace. "Your sense of peace comes from the power of those prayers." He paused for a moment. "You have so many people praying for you, you don't even need to pray for yourself."

Something went up my arm. I was silent, sitting on the sofa in his office, absorbing his words. I tried to concentrate on being in the moment, aware of what was happening, aware of the power. As I write this, I am trying to reconstruct a formula, hoping to remember when it is the next person's turn, how to pass it on.

For now, while I still have your attention, keep the prayers coming this way. How can I just say thank you?

Hugs, Sigourney

My spirits lift at the thought of my message instantly reaching eighty friends, but the responses make me soar. There is an honesty, a sacredness in the words I read. Mary Ann writes back:

Do you know how much we would all love to feel and see the world from the perspective you describe? . . . we take living in such love and beauty for granted—once the possibility of it not being there is ripped from our soul, the life and love of our family take on such color and texture . . . thank you for helping me jump in deep with life where I am.

Cathy, a cancer survivor from California, writes about meditation:

SILENCE CAN BE AN INTIMIDATING REQUIREMENT WHEN YOUR MIND AND HEART ARE OVERCROWDED WITH CONCERNS AND ARE WORKING OVERTIME. BREAKING THROUGH TO A COMFORTABLE SILENCE CAN TAKE A LITTLE WHILE. PERSEVERE. IT IS WORTH IT.

Alice writes:

YOU HAVE FOUND YOUR VOICE. YOUR DETAILS ARE AS WELL-CHOSEN AS THE OBJECTS IN YOUR DRAWING ROOM.

Kathy writes:

GOD IS GOOD TO US. HE ALLOWS OUR SUFFERING, BUT OFFERS PEACE AND BLESSINGS THAT FLOW THROUGH THE LOVE AND CARE OF OTHERS. YOU WILL BE CHANGED FOREVER.

Anne Taylor is:

INSPIRED BY SPENDING A GOODLY PORTION OF THE DAY WITH YOU IN THE TREATMENT ROOM . . . AND WITNESSING . . . A KIND OF BOLDNESS AND FORTHRIGHT BELIEF IN WHAT MY FRIENDS AND THEIR CARING CAN DO FOR ME.

Life Is Rich

As days pass, I continue to receive notes and flowers and books. Robin gives me Mary Oliver's *Why I Wake Early*, and I think of grappling with life's mysteries as I read the first three lines of the poem, "Where Does the Temple Begin, Where Does It End?":

> There are things you can't reach.
> But you can reach out to them, and all day long.
> The wind, the bird flying away. The idea of God.

As difficult as it is to grapple with the possible consequences of cancer, something rich is growing from this new view of the world.

I walk with my trainer, Janet, on Wednesday afternoons. Before the diagnosis, we met twice a week, once at the gym to work on the machines and once at my house to exercise with free weights and walk, but I've cut the workout to once a week for a while. She has been working to improve my muscle tone and stamina for over six years, and over that time we have developed a special friendship, sharing life's intimacies as I pump iron and perform "pre-ski" lunges. She adds a twist to my meditation story. She read about a Buddhist meditation practice of breathing in all the wrongs of the world and releasing goodness and healing. I imagine hundreds, no thousands, no millions of people practicing this technique.

Even though I have put my volunteer life on hold, I want to go to the YWCA board meeting in late May. My friend and cousin, Donna, who is married to another Cheek, is retiring as director. My friend, Patricia, is retiring as director of development. We have worked together over the last few years, and I want to be there to wish them well and godspeed. Donna brought us dinner a few weeks ago and mentioned she had shared my e-mails with various staff people and board members and hoped that was OK. I didn't think much about the sharing until I walked into the boardroom. After my absence of a few months, instead of people not knowing what to say, many give me hugs. Donna's passing on of the e-mails made most of the group familiar with details of my diagnosis, and no one was afraid to approach me, to tell me they were thinking of me, praying for me, to share another cancer or recovery story.

As I articulate the day-to-day challenges of my disease one e-mail at a time, the mysteries of dealing with cancer unfold in pieces easier to digest. My e-mail contacts increase each time I send another message. At last count, the list is up to one hundred. I awaken each morning and open new responses that touch my heart.

A YWCA staff member, Jan, approaches me at the end of the board meeting. She shares with me her own close encounter with death, a car accident several years ago. The doctors gave her a 10 percent chance of moving her legs, less chance to walk. She inspires me. I must put her story in my heart to share in the next e-mail. Jan asks to be added to my list and begins to send beautifully articulated responses that I open with ever-increasing enthusiasm and comfort as a friendship grows with a woman I have known, but haven't really known, for six years.

Back to the Beach

⁓

*T*he next Ponte Vedra trip is planned for Memorial Day weekend. Jim and I are excited about a large crowd: Jamie and Lisa and Jack and Baker; Lisa's mom, Nancy; and Grandpa Jim. That includes four Jim Cheeks: Grandpa, husband, son, and grandson. Pretty special. Middle son, Daniel, is also there with his girlfriend, Anne. Daniel met Anne last year at a party in Columbus where he is doing his emergency-room medical residency. The timing of our beach party, right before the second chemo, will be when I have the most energy to enjoy a full house. Just as advertised, the fatigue peaks after each treatment, and strength builds back over the three weeks before the next chemo. Then I start a round again.

The best part of the weekend is being with the babies. At three months old and two years old, they don't notice a grandma who can't keep up. Baker spends an hour on a beach towel under a big umbrella. Jack fills his bucket with water, digs a hole that fills with more water, and finds a starfish that he carries around for the rest of the day. Jamie catches a baby shark and throws it back. The freezer is taken over by plastic bags of sandy squid bait, and half the fridge is filled with a variety of beers, but I vow not to complain. The toys I am falling over in the living room are part of the package that comes with enjoying my two precious grandchildren. We have bought Jack a toy that drops three balls down a funnel and through a chute and tosses them up again to the top while playing accordion-like musical tunes over and over. Jack can keep track of those balls and send them down the chute over and over and isn't he clever and can't his father and uncle make less of a mess so there is some order left in our confined living space? Jack is the reincarnation of Jamie at the same age, his personality still unfolding, all possibilities holding only promise and delight.

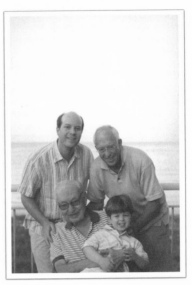

The four James Cheeks at the beach.

We eat peel-'em-and-eat-'em shrimp using my mother's recipe: Dump shrimp into heavy pot and cover with son's beer and a crab-seasoning bag and marinate for a few hours. Make a salad and heat crusty bread while the temperature slowly rises under the shrimp. Stir 'til they come to a boil and turn pink. Remove immediately, drain, and eat. (The key is to be brave, be firm, and as soon as they boil, serve. If they sit or boil too long, they get mushy—trust me, not what you want.) Serve with the homemade tomato-based shrimp sauce from your local fish market. If you insist, also serve with melted butter and lemon, but talk about fattening.

Wouldn't you rather save the calories for ice cream? Your choice—and remember to let the kids do the dishes.

On Sunday, after the morning on the beach, I wash my hair and glance down on the white-tile

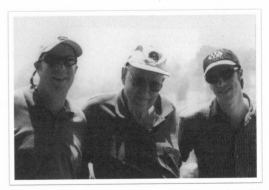

Jamie, Grandpa, and Daniel.

floor as I blow it dry. Panic. There are hairs all over the floor. Short, black threads are visible against the white tiles. My God, it's happening. Three weeks after the first chemo, my locks are beginning to shed. I put down the dryer, stop combing, start sweeping.

To add to the bad news, coming home on the plane on Monday, I have a sore throat. Tuesday and Wednesday, I have a slight fever. I know my immune system is compromised by the leukemia. I sit under the covers in bed, feeling miserable, collecting hair off my pillow and my white pajama top, and trying to calculate the amount of time it will take for the rest of my hair to fall and how my flu symptoms will play out under the mantle of my disease. I spread my fingers through my hair to keep it off my face, and a small clump comes off in my hand. I wonder if I got my money's worth from the pixie cut. Yeah, those compliments were the best.

Connie and I went to the Nashville Hair Prosthesis place in Bellevue right before the first chemo. They cut a piece of my hair for an exact match. We decided to go a little lighter, as dark hair seems to look harsh when you start to color it to disguise grey, and wouldn't a wig be the same? The wig lady told me for cancer patients, the wig can be ready in two days. I paid 50 percent down and was assured that I could be reimbursed if I am one of the small percent who doesn't lose her hair. A nice lady at Vanderbilt gave me a free wig, a hat, and some scarves during the first chemo session. I could have made do, but it was kind of like those expensive shoes in New York.

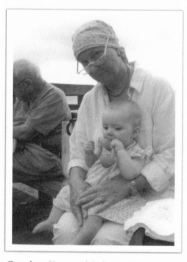

Grandpa, Siggy, and Baker in Monteagle.

Back in Nashville, before I succumb to bed and sore throat, I make time to fire off the next e-mail.

UPDATE FROM PATIENT SIGGY
MONDAY, JUNE 6, 2005
DEAR FRIENDS,

EACH TIME I SEND AN UPDATE, I ADD A DOZEN-PLUS NAMES TO THE LIST. I AM HAPPY THAT PEOPLE WANT TO BE INCLUDED. THEY ARE SAYING, "I WANT TO LISTEN, I CARE." MAYBE THAT'S WHAT PRAYER IS, PEOPLE WHO ARE THINKING OF YOU, ONCE A DAY OR SO, OFFERING YOUR NAME, WITH OTHERS, TO A POWER BEYOND THEMSELVES.

LAST WEEK, WE HAD A WONDERFUL MEMORIAL DAY WEEKEND IN PONTE VEDRA WITH MOST OF OUR FAMILY, INCLUDING TWO-YEAR-OLD JACK AND THREE-MONTH-OLD BAKER, GRAND-MOTHERS NANCY AND ME, GREAT-GRANDPA JIM, AS WELL AS THE TWO JIMS IN-BETWEEN, JIM AND JAMIE, AND DANIEL AND HIS NEW GIRLFRIEND, ANNE. THE BEACH WAS PERFECT ENOUGH TO TAKE BAKER DOWN FOR A FEW HOURS NOW AND THEN. WE WALKED THE BEACH,

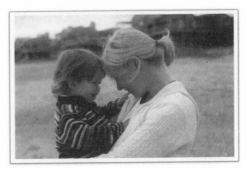

Lisa and Jack.

ATE SEAFOOD, PEEL-'EM-AND-EAT-'EM SHRIMP TWICE, WE LAUGHED. JACK FOUND A STARFISH AND CARRIED IT AROUND FOR THE REST OF THE DAY. JAMIE CAUGHT A BABY SHARK.

THEN ON SUNDAY I WASHED, BLEW-DRY MY HAIR AND USED MY NEW "CHE" HAIR-CURLER THING, TRYING TO FLIP UP THE SIDES OF MY SHORT DO, AND A LOCK STAYED ON THE CURLER. I LOOKED DOWN AT THE WHITE BATHROOM FLOOR AND RAN TO THE CLOSET FOR THE BROOM AND DUST PAN. MONDAY I HAD A SORE THROAT AND TRIED NOT TO TOUCH MY HAIR. TUESDAY I HAD A FEVER. I SPENT THE DAY IN BED AND WATCHED THE HAIR ACCUMULATE ON MY PILLOW. I FINALLY HAD TO WASH IT. I KEPT A FOOT ON THE SHOWER DRAIN TO PREVENT YOU-KNOW-WHAT FROM CLOGGING.

When I dried my head, one side of the white towel was black. A call to the nurse practitioner confirmed it would be OK to go ahead with the chemo on Friday as I didn't appear to have a secondary infection. She said my hair would be gone in a few days and recommended going ahead and shaving it off. I looked in the mirror. It was thin but I still had a full head of hair. I couldn't face her suggestion. Plus, I felt like shit. Connie and I had gone to the wig place last week to be measured for a spiffy wig. The woman said to call when I started to lose my hair. I did. I decided that I needed to get through the weekend. I wouldn't see anyone anyway. The place is closed on Monday. My appointment for shave and wig is Tuesday.

The hardest part of this challenge is the diagnosis and rediagnosis, from B-cell lymphoma, to CLL, to Richter's syndrome (which is really a transformation into a B-cell lymphoma so I guess all of the diagnoses were on the money.) I try to wrap around all of this information to figure out what it means. I didn't even know what leukemia or lymphoma really meant. Even after reading dozens of articles, I am still confused. In a way, an even harder part is the hair. No matter how many people say, "it's just hair, it will grow back," I don't care. Women, vanity, the historical significance of cutting a woman's hair off, I think about all of these things. Mary Jane came over with dinner the other night and agreed that, for her, the hair loss was the hardest part.

Enough complaining. I read an essay in an American Cancer Society magazine in which a woman describes how she felt when diagnosed with cancer, "I remember how utterly surprised I was when I noticed that longtime friends and associates looked at me differently, as though I was already gone. A stranger to my friends and increasingly on my own, my very identity was dissolving." If I knew her number, I would call her and say, "Honey, we need to talk." My experience has been just the opposite. The more I try to learn and embrace the challenge and call on God's help and pull on the power of all of my friends who surround me, I feel miracles happening and power bouncing between all of us.

Reading the letters and e-mails, and listening to special conversations are such a gift.

I haven't been doing much volunteering, but I went to the last YW Board meeting last week because Donna Cheek is retiring. She had brought dinner one night last week and told me that she had passed on my e-mails to staff members who knew me. When I arrived, instead of people being apprehensive, they were familiar with where I was and embracing.

Jan, a staff member, told me that she had put me in her prayer box. My expression conveyed to Jan that I wanted to know more. She told me about her car accident. She woke up paralyzed from the neck down. The doctors gave her a 10% chance to move again. She is a tall, slender redhead. She now walks gracefully with only a slight limp. No cane. The trauma and recovery changed her life. She now keeps a small Shaker box. She has written the names of the people she prays for on individual pieces of paper. She takes the names out, fingers them, as she prays for each person. I don't think she would have shared this sacred part of her life without having read my e-mails. I didn't know her very well. Now I do. I'm looking for a small box and some beautiful handmade paper.

Responding to my e-mails Cathy wrote:

> There are so many sweet blessings that come about with having cancer. Truthfully, I gained much more than I had to suffer, and life, friends, and my family all are part of what I treasure most now. God is good to us. He allows our suffering, but offers peace and blessings that flow through the love and care of others. You will be changed forever.

Randy wrote:

> I have come up with the answer to an eternal, heretofore unanswered question that has haunted humanity forever: Why do women live longer than men? It's simple: You girls stick together. When one of you is down, the herd comes to the rescue.

Mary Ann wrote:

It really is inside of a full and alive circle that we exist. We give, we love, we care, we worry, and what we put out there comes back around and circles and intersects with what others love, care about, worry about, and what they put out there in the world . . . such a beautiful life.

Becca wrote:

My prayers and all the prayers from every service at the chapel continue to fill the skies.

There are so many beautiful writers out there. And on my front step this morning was a hand-crafted Shaker box. A gift from Jan. Now all I need is special paper.

Hugs to all of you and please keep those powerful prayers and words coming.

Hugs, Sigourney

I think a lot about the woman who felt as if she had disappeared since her diagnosis with breast cancer. That girl needs to discover e-mails. Sharing my story has let people know I don't mind talking about my illness, and the feedback is a constant source of nourishment.

Jan responds immediately to the e-mail:

Thank you for including me in your distribution list. This is a gift to be able to walk with you through this journey. I know it is a bumpy road and I am sorry that you have to walk it. You are truly blessed to have so many loved ones walking with you.

I am glad you like the Shaker box. W.C. (Willola) Tyson made it. She lives in Clinton, Tennessee, and comes to the TACA fair, the Tennessee Association of Craft Artists. I have a small collection of Shaker boxes and started using one like the one I gave you several years ago as my prayer box. As I have held and handled my box over the years, the

CHERRY HAS DARKENED AND THE BOX SEEMS TO HAVE A SPECIAL ENERGY ALL ITS OWN. LOTS OF GOOD THINGS AND POSITIVE ENERGY HAVE SURROUNDED IT, LO THESE MANY YEARS, THAT'S FOR SURE. I SO APPRECIATE THE RITUAL OF READING A MORNING MEDITATION AND HOLDING THE BOX IN MY LAP. I DUMP THE NAMES IN THE LID, AND AS I PRAY FOR EACH ONE, I PLACE THEM BACK IN THE BOX, PUT THE LID BACK ON, FEEL THE WOOD OF THE BOX, AND PLACE IT BACK ON THE TABLE.

AS WE DISCUSSED, MY PRAYER FOR YOU EACH DAY (AND OFTEN WHEN I AWAKE AT NIGHT, IT SO HAPPENS) CONTINUES TO BE FOR PEACE (THAT SURPASSES ALL UNDERSTANDING), THAT YOU WILL BE ABLE TO TOLERATE THE MEDS REASONABLY WELL, AND THAT YOU MAY BE ABLE TO FIND THE GLIMMER OF LIGHT EACH DAY AND WHATEVER MEANING IS TO BE FOUND IN THE JOURNEY. AS EVIDENCED BY YOUR WRITINGS, YOU HAVE AN AMAZING CAPACITY TO WATCH, LISTEN, LEARN, AND EXPERIENCE GRATITUDE.

I HOPE TODAY IS A GOOD DAY FOR YOU AND THAT YOUR WEEKEND BRINGS SOME LAUGHTER AND JOY.

PEACE.

Dr. Greer's nurse practitioner, Ellen, tells me about a man with CLL who had it for ten years and had been in the hospital on multiple occasions for various treatments including chemo. He would go right back to work and never tell a soul. He didn't want anyone to know about his condition. Shoot, if I'm going to be sick, I want the attention; no, more than that, I feed on the attention.

An anonymous quote I heard the other day puts it another way: "Most of us can run all day on one good compliment."

Ellen confirms the go-ahead for the second chemo on Friday, scheduled three weeks after the first one. I do have a bad cold, but she feels there are no signs of a secondary infection so we can still go ahead with the treatment. She also confirms that I should call the wig place and set the appointment to have the rest of my hair shaved off, but I can't make the call, especially feeling so shitty. An attempt at deep breathing into my diaphragm only makes me cough. I can't fathom doing this tomorrow. I am sick and Jim is out of town for the whole week. Finally I manage to make the appointment for hair removal. I can always cancel. On the phone, the lady tells me they will shampoo my hair and then shave my head. They can turn the chair away from the mirror so I don't have to watch. Whoopee. I take it back about wanting to be in this movie. I hope the director is still around and will yell, "Cut." Connie calls to check on me. She agrees to take me to the wig place the Tuesday after the second chemo, giving me a small iota of peace of mind.

Mary Jane brings supper and I give her the hair report. As she is sharing her own cancer experiences, I realize I didn't pay enough attention to her when she was going through the early stages of her disease. I make a note to be more attentive to others who are diagnosed in the future and try not to be too hard on myself. Only those who have been through cancer understand the healing power of the cancer sisterhood.

Chemo Two

$\mathcal{T}$he second chemo, on June 3, is easier than the first. The chemos are scheduled for every three weeks and I have chosen Fridays, so I have the weekend to recover with Jim at home to help. The day of chemo starts again with blood drawn and analyzed to assure counts are high enough to proceed. Many patients have to wait more than three weeks between treatments to build up blood counts or have a transfusion before the next round. My white blood count is up slightly. But unlike many leukemia patients, blood-count irregularities are still not a serious issue with my disease. I am familiar now with the lineup of drugs for my CHOP+R cocktail. I have been given written material on each of the drugs and their possible side effects. I skim the information, but choose not to dwell on side effects unless they occur. I figure I have enough to worry about without the anticipation of symptoms I may never see.

The hospital world exists on its own schedule, giving me lots of time to think. Asking about the time to allow for a given procedure I again hear, "Oh, about forty-five minutes, but I would allow a couple of hours." You wouldn't sit in a lawyer's office for an hour before an appointment, but doctors' days are filled with unexpected emergencies, like the day of my diagnosis when I was one of the unscheduled patients who spent most of the day in the examination room. Now I arrive at the hospital and no longer worry about the time it will take. I will be there for a while, always. My other world has stopped anyway. I understand how people can become isolated with this disease. Without Carole's food brigade, without Connie's hospital helpers, without my e-mail group, I would be isolated too.

Ellen comes down from her office on the second floor to the chemo area on the first. I am settled into my lounge chair in one of the eight-by-ten foot chemo rooms. We haven't really had a chance to eyeball each other, and I appreciate her visit. She gives me a prescription for trazodone to replace Ambien, which, she tells me, will lose its effectiveness if taken over an extended period of time. She sees me make notes in my journal, my marble notebook, and claims that statistics show that people who journal about their cancer have a better recovery rate. When Ellen leaves, I ask my friends sitting with me about their spin on prayer. Carole H. thinks if you are thinking of a person with positive thoughts, you are praying for them. Anne Taylor describes many photos of family on her fridge and the kind thoughts that pass through her mind each time she looks at them as she opens the door.

Time passes quickly with such good company throughout the long day. I think of the burden of being the caregiver, a task more difficult than being the patient. Yet with so many caregivers, maybe it will not be too great a burden on any one of them.

I am home at five. I sit for a minute on the side porch and watch the mother robin fly into the nest to feed her babies, watch the father scolding from the crepe myrtle near the bird bath, angry at me for invading his temporary home. I walk up to the garden by the pool and stop in front of a large clump of hot-pink silla. Two bees are busy darting from one tiny flower to the next, extracting pollen that I can see being collected in small yellow clusters under their bodies. They move efficiently from one stem to another. I wonder how far they will travel to the hive to turn the pollen dust into honey, which I use to sweeten my green tea each morning instead of the artificial sweeteners with aspartame. I remembered a spring wildflower walk last year deep in the woods of Monteagle Mountain. I remember taking time to kneel down and look at a tiny wildflower the size of my pinky finger through a jeweler's loop. I remember the intricacy of the design, the ranges of blue and yellow in the center of the flower, details undetected by the human eye alone. I remember thinking of the millions upon millions of tiny flowers in the woods in spring that open with equally exquisite petals and stamen and pollen and have no audience to admire them except the bees. My old life was usually too busy for such reflection. Now I inhabit a suspended world, where the ordinary rhythms of my old life and the interaction with the outside world are no longer important. I'm savoring the warm evening, the anticipation of the next friend who wants to visit my side porch, and always the flowers surrounding me.

We are supposed to go to a wedding in the Carolinas, but the long drive is too daunting to consider. I will hear the reports from my bed on Sunday.

On June 6, the Monday following last Friday's chemo, I return to the doctor's office for a routine white-blood booster shot, Neulasta. Regardless of the blood counts, all chemo patients receive this shot forty-eight hours after chemo to build back the cells that have been zapped.

In the waiting room I run into Nancy and Alan, a couple I know. Jim and I actually ran into them last week at a reception for the new president of the Cheekwood Botanical Garden and Museum of Art in Nashville. OK, I cheated. I'm not supposed to be going to big gatherings. But the museum is one of my passions and the new president, Jack, is the best president in my thirty-plus years of involvement, and besides, we only stayed for an hour. The reception was packed and I don't remember how we got onto the subject at the party, but Alan told me he had just been diagnosed with myloma and his doctor was Dr. Greer. We compared notes. I know his wife is a breast-cancer survivor. There must be a cancer radar alerting one pilgrim to seek another. I am keeping a record of couples who share cancer.

I am glad Alan is also a patient of Dr. Greer, and we swap war stories in the waiting room. His wife talks about reading everything she could when she was diagnosed with her cancer, and she turns to her husband and says, "He has to start reading about his disease." I see a look of overload on his face that mirrored my own reaction when Jim was telling me the same thing. I smile at her and say, "You are the reader in your family. Jim is doing the reading for me." The expression on her husband's face lightens.

He also shares the trauma of the scales, the surprise over his weight. I tell him about my scale boycott, and I know by his smile that he will soon join my rebel team.

As I become comfortable with the rhythms of my disease, I listen to stories from people who devour every word they can on their illness. You don't even need to go to the library. Just click on the Internet and you can scan articles for hours. Jim had a hip replacement several years ago as well as the prostrate surgery last year. If there is any research available on either subject that he has not read, I would be surprised. I remember the day he brought home the book on prostate cancer that was two inches thick. Sometimes I think he is fulfilling early yearnings. (I struggled through a required science course as a freshman in college while Jim, at one point, was a pre-med student at Duke.) I was confident I had the best doctor in Nashville, and I'd even had a consultation with the other choice for number one. Dr. John and Dr. Bill and Dr. Roy were all close enough friends to be part of the group coming with me to Mallorca for my birthday celebration. I was surrounded by impressive medical minds. I would focus on my journal and leave the reading to Jim and the doctor team.

In the first few weeks of diagnosis, when Jim and I would meet with Dr. Greer, he would always suggest a range of treatments and options of chemo doses and meds. He would tell us the other top specialists he had consulted and only then offer his best advice. It took me until now to get it. Because my type of cancer did not require immediate action, I didn't start chemo until a month after diagnosis, allowing lots of tests and lots of consulting and lots of digesting of options to happen before being zapped with one of the heaviest doses of chemo available. I needed to read the basics to have some understanding of leukemia and lymphoma and even the dreaded Richter's syndrome, but the information I gained from the reading would not be sufficient to determine the path of treatment. My reading would only help offset the fear of the unknown.

Baldy

*T*omorrow, June 7, four days after the second chemo, three weeks and four days after the first chemo, I am scheduled to have the rest of my hair shaved away. There is so little left that I have a scarf on in Dr. Greer's office. I am ready. I have dealt long enough with hair removal from my pillow, my clothes, my mind. I didn't even try to wash it when I took a shower this morning: too many consequences, and besides, it will be gone tomorrow.

Anne and Connie pick me up Tuesday morning for the trip to the Hair Prosthesis Institute and head-shaving. I tell them they can stay in the waiting room, but the troopers both come into the room with me. I did turn away from the mirror in my swivel chair, but they watched and talked to me as I was being sheared, our friendship moving into another dimension.

For about six years, Connie and Anne and I worked full-time. We rented a large shop that housed our antiques business. Road trips were spent gathering treasures and finds that passed too briefly through our hands, cramming our car or rental van with the 1930s painting of the girl with a riding crop—which I'm still sorry I sold—or the 1880s aesthetic-movement slipper chair. But the memories remain to be cherished.

I still hold fond memories of the first time we went on the road with dealer friends, Randy and Michael, to a wholesale antiques market in Atlanta called Scotts. The first night we stayed at the same seedy motel together, awoke at 5:00 AM the next day to position for a first pick of the merchandise. We were still loading purchases in the back of our station wagon at 7:00 PM. I called the Ritz Carlton on my cell phone, booked a room, ordered room service, and we took turns soaking in the oversized tub. We needed to assimilate low-budget travel a little at a time. Connie slept in the extra roll-away bed. Connie always sleeps in the smaller bed in the hotel rooms we share. She's so little. She says she's five feet, but don't believe it. Her vibrant, edgy personality makes up for it. Anne, on the other hand, is very tall, reed thin, and graceful. Her hair is usually in perfect order, her nails are always manicured. Her voice and manner espouse Southern hospitality. When Connie's and my Yankee edges start to cut, Anne forms a buffer and tension soon subsides. We went on subsequent trips to England and France, and specialized in unique, iron light fixtures from the Paris flea market. What a ride.

Now we have downsized to a large room in a building filled with antiques dealers where we pay the rent and they take care of all the sales and customer issues. The timing of the downsizing couldn't be better for me. I wouldn't want to be handling the day-to-day issues of a shop. Starting and running a business was an unforgettable adventure. Add to the memory mix Anne and Connie witnessing the shaving of my head. I will love them forever.

In the three weeks after the second chemo, I cancel another invitation, a planned trip to Destin with Jamie, Lisa, the babies, and the rest of Lisa's family. So many people in the same house seems overwhelming. I cancel an invitation to a society ball. We do go to the smaller dinner for big donors, and I wear my wig and my smashing Zoran outfit from New York. The compliments from around the room are over the top. Is it the cancer, the sympathy, or am I just a sensational old broad? Who cares? I have a great time, and the photograph in the local society rag makes me look great.

I usually thrive on the party scene, but the two recent outings exhaust me. For now, I need to allow my world to revolve around home and my garden and to relish the peace. Alice comes one afternoon. We listen to Joan Baez and she gives me a reflexology foot massage with three different lotions. Alice is another person whose friendship started with writing. She has published several books and offers advice to help me move forward from journaling to writing that can be passed on. Lou Anne, who shares volunteer jobs with me, drops off a huge bouquet of Casablanca lilies from the ball I missed. They smell delicious and last for over a week on the table in front of the living-room window.

I try to walk each morning. I watch Jack in our pool in late afternoon jumping from the raft to his father's arms, and in my journal I try to record the richness of each moment, the magic of this new life, the sacredness of the ordinary.

More Spiritual Ammunition

I meet with Ken each week. I assume daily meditation will become part of my routine after the euphoria I felt from it before the first chemo, but this has not happened. I want to go to the keyboard, not a quiet, silent place. Have I really changed? I talk to Ken and tell him I am not in the same place as I was before the first chemo, with a constant awareness of God with me on the journey. The immediacy of His presence has dimmed, although I know He is still with me. A sense of peace still surrounds me. My blood pressure is still down. The lump under my arm is still gone.

Ken says, "It's better to be in the place where you are now, because this is reality." I tell him I have been reading over past journals from his classes in 2000 on spiritual direction. In one series of exercises, we reviewed the seven deadly sins, the subject of some of Ken's best sermons. He has a chilling way of making each one about me instead of that guy over there. I did a lot of journaling then, recognizing myself in all of those sins. But somehow now, as I read over my jottings of each sin one-by-one, I realize that for me, at the moment, sin is not an issue on the table. I ask Ken to explain why I feel disconnected with wrongdoings. He explains that sin is for ordinary lives when we become self-absorbed in our own agenda, each desire, each disappointment. At least for a short moment, that part of my life is on hold. Sin is for well people.

Two of the bug bites that were a constant affliction before the first chemo have returned. I am scratching again under my left chin and returning to the remedy drawer for salves. I look in the mirror and see the white circles, or lesions. Their appearance is a discouraging sign. The doctors never confirmed that the bug bites had a

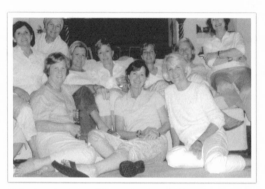
Friends gathering on Monteagle Moutain for Linda's birthday.

direct relationship to my cancer, but I knew that they did. An exaggerated reaction to bug bites is a classic symptom of CLL. In my case, the initial swelling of the bug site expanded to the size of an egg. I am convinced that the infected bites caused the lymph nodes to swell and alerted me to a diagnosis of cancer earlier than I would otherwise have experienced. But why the bites would return after they had completely disappeared disturbs me. The bug bites were back. Did that mean the lumps under my arms would soon be back?

I am distracted by a few gatherings with close friends. Two days before my next chemo, eight women gather on the top of Monteagle Mountain, some at Carole's mountain home, some at Nicky's, to celebrate Linda's sixtieth birthday. A surprising number of our friends have invested in second homes on the mountain, the home of Sewanee, the University of the South. The sacredness of our inner circle of friends looms large at tonight's gathering as it did at Anne and John's dinner. We sit around a big table in Carole's living room and laugh about the quirks of aging, but I look around and think we are not a bad-looking group. I wear my scarf. The expensive wig is too hot. It's lined with plastic. What were they thinking? Two other members of the group are cancer survivors, both veterans of hair loss. Another had breast surgery after one biopsy too many. At the end of the evening, we talk about the next birthday. All have been invited for my sixtieth birthday celebration in Mallorca in August.

Explosion

The next day I return home from the mountain and hit the keyboard. Each e-mail seems to spill forth more easily than the last.

UPDATE FROM PATIENT SIGGY
JUNE 23, 2005
DEAR FRIENDS,

THE HEAT HAS MADE THE OCCASIONAL COOLER DAY A GIFT. THE TIME IS EARLY MORNING, AND I AM WRITING ON MY LAPTOP ON MY SIDE PORCH. THE TEMPERATURE IS IN THE LOW 70S. THE MORNING LIGHT SPREADS ACROSS THE SPRING GRASS, THE BLADES BENDING TO THE RIGHT, TO THE LEFT, UNDECIDED.

GREEN DOMINATES THE GARDEN, BETWEEN SPRING AND SUMMER BLOOM. DOZENS OF HOSTAS ARE EACH A DIFFERENT SHADE OF GREEN, THE LAMB'S EAR ANOTHER, THE HOLLYHOCK LEAVES ANOTHER. THE ONLY COLOR COMES FROM THE LAST FOXGLOVE, A FEW ADENOPHORA, AND THE EMERGING NASTURTIUMS, INCHING TO THE EDGE OF THE EIGHTEEN-INCH RETAINING WALL WHERE BY JULY THEY WILL CASCADE DOWN AND TOUCH THE GRASS BELOW. THE FOUNTAIN SPILLS GENTLY INTO THE POOL AS TWO ROBINS HAVE A CONVERSATION, ONE IN THE MAPLE TO THE LEFT OF ME, THE OTHER IN THE CREPE MYRTLE ON MY RIGHT.

THE PRACTICE OF BEING IN THE MOMENT STARTS EASILY HERE. MY CALENDAR IS BLANK. I HAVE WIPED OUT THE RITUALS OF MY LIFE. I HAVE DECLINED ALL INVITATIONS FOR COMMUNITY BOARD MEETINGS, PARTIES FOR CAUSES, FUNCTIONS FOR JIM'S BUSINESS INTERESTS. MY WORLD HAS STOPPED AND GOOD STUFF IS SURFACING IN THE STILLNESS LEFT BEHIND.

WHY DO WE WAIT FOR THE FACE OF DEATH TO PASS OVER US LIKE A SHADOW TO HAVE AN I/THOU CONVERSATION WITH TEN FRIENDS? WHY DO WE HAVE TO BE ILL TO TAKE TIME TO VISIT WITH

AN INSPIRATIONAL NINETY-YEAR-OLD COUSIN WHO IS A SIX-YEAR CANCER SURVIVOR? I SPEND TIME WONDERING, WHEN THIS IS OVER, AND I HOPE IT WILL BE OVER, WILL I GO BACK? REYNOLDS PRICE PUTS IT SO WELL IN HIS BOOK ON ILLNESS AND HEALING, *A Whole New Life*, "REYNOLDS PRICE IS DEAD. WHO WILL YOU BE NOW?"

THE INITIAL EUPHORIA BEFORE THE FIRST CHEMO HAS PASSED, BUT I CONTINUE TO BE SURROUNDED BY A COVER OF PEACE FROM THE CONSTANT AFFIRMATION FROM FRIENDS WHO ARE THINKING OF ME, PRAYING FOR ME, SHARING THEIR OWN TRIALS. I KNOW I AM UNIQUELY BLESSED BY THE CONSTANT CALLS, NOTES, AND DINNERS. I WISH EVERYONE WHO EXPERIENCED CANCER HAD THIS SAME ATTENTION, BUT I KNOW THEY DO NOT. I AM HUMBLED BY THIS GIFT.

WRITING THESE E-MAILS HAS BEEN A BRIDGE TO SO MANY FRIENDS. MY COMMENTS ABOUT HAIR LOSS HAVE SOLICITED THE MOST RESPONSES FROM THOSE WHO HAVE ALSO EXPERIENCED IT. ONE FRIEND DROVE IN A CONVERTIBLE, WITH A GLASS OF WINE, AND PULLED HER HAIR OUT, TOSSING IT TO THE WIND. ONE FRIEND HAD HAD IT AND ASKED HER HUSBAND TO SHAVE OFF WHAT WAS LEFT AND THEN WAITED AS EACH OF HER THREE CHILDREN REACTED DIFFERENTLY FROM TEARS TO LAUGHTER ABOUT HER CHANGED APPEARANCE. ONE FRIEND STOOD AT THE KITCHEN SINK, LET THE WATER RUN AND PULLED OUT PIECE AFTER PIECE TO FILL THE SINK.

I WENT TO THE HAIR PROSTHESIS INSTITUTE IN BELLEVUE WITH CONNIE AND ANNE AND THEY WATCHED, I DIDN'T, AS THE THIRD OF HAIR THAT WAS LEFT WAS SHAVED OFF BY ONE OF THE STAFF AND MY NEW WIG WAS FITTED AND CUT. EVERYONE SAYS THE WIG LOOKS FINE, BUT IT'S HOT AND I HAVE TURNED INTO NATHAN LANE IN *The Birdcage*.

THE FIRST NIGHT WITH MY NEW DO (OR IS IT UNDO?), I WOKE ABOUT THREE AND WENT INTO THE BATHROOM. I WONDERED HOW THE CAT HAD GOTTEN OUT OF THE KITCHEN AND WAS SITTING ON THE SINK. THEN I LOOKED AGAIN AND IT WAS MY WIG.

THERE ARE DECIDEDLY SOME NO-HAIR PERKS; MAYBE DAVID LETTERMAN WOULD BE INTERESTED:

1. *Fifteen extra minutes per day for something else*
2. *No bad hair days*

3. *An opportunity to look dramatic in a selection of scarves*
4. *An opportunity to wear big hats and not be labeled a drama queen*
5. *Few hair-house expenses except initial wig trim which will require no retrim in six weeks*
6. *Wig stays clean, set, and combed while sitting on my other styrofoam head as I sleep*
7. *Shower time is down to two minutes*
8. *I have a short wig, a long wig, one of mine is magenta and I'm thinking about adding blond*
9. *When Jim wants to drive with the top down it's no longer a problem*
10. *If I decided to streak it, I can just drop it off, or better yet, send it in a taxi*

My next chemo, number three, is tomorrow. The drill has become routine. Anne and Marcella will keep me company and I know we will laugh. How about a green wig as a tribute to my garden?

Thank you all for the continuous love.

Hugs, Sigourney

Within an hour the responses start filling my inbox:

Mary writes:

When you lose your hair, accept the loss of vanity, you're just getting closer to the real you—the Sigourney inside—the part that really matters to everyone who knows and cares for you.

Cancer survivor Cathy adds:

And yes, the hair part is horrible . . . It is the neon sign that says "I have cancer."

Becca writes:

As I rush to get all of my e-mails this morning before I start the endless task of trying to keep house in order with

THREE BOYS . . . YOU HAVE MADE ME STOP. I AM DEAD IN MY TRACKS.
I FEEL LIKE TAKING MY FIRST STEP OF THE DAY. PLEASE KEEP ME ON
YOUR LIST AND SINCE YOU ARE WALKING CLOSE TO GOD, PLEASE
TELL GOD HELLO FROM WAY OUT HERE. I AM LOVING YOU.

Becca, a cross between ethereal and earthy with long, flowing hair, happens to be an Episcopal priest. I am absorbed by her words. I think about a person who has devoted her life to serving God perceiving me as having an inside track. And then I remember that until you have a close encounter with death, you cannot walk the path I walk. I still hold death in my hand, and it is a frightening yet holy place.

Jan writes:

I'LL BE THINKING ABOUT YOU TODAY AS YOU GET YOUR DRIP
. . . I KNOW FROM EXPERIENCE WHAT A DIFFERENCE IT MAKES
THAT PEOPLE ARE LIFTING YOU UP EACH DAY—PEOPLE YOU
DON'T EVEN KNOW. I AGREE THAT IT IS TOO BAD THAT WE
OFTEN DON'T PAY ATTENTION TO THE IMPORTANT STUFF UNTIL
IT IS THREATENED TO BE TAKEN AWAY. I DO BELIEVE GOD IS
WITH US MOST WHEN WE ARE MOST VULNERABLE BECAUSE WE
OPEN OURSELVES UP TO BE RECEIVED—AND IT COMES FROM
EVERYWHERE DOESN'T IT?

THANKS FOR SHARING YOUR MORNING GARDEN EXPERIENCE
FROM THE SIDE PORCH PERSPECTIVE . . . THE NASTURTIUM CRANING
THEIR NECKS TOWARDS THE LIGHT. KIND OF LIKE WE DO ON THE
SPIRITUAL JOURNEY, HUH?

Beth, a journalist, writes:

FINDING YOUR BEAUTIFUL E-MAIL LAST NIGHT, I WAS SO MOVED. AS
YOU FEEL BLESSED BY OTHERS' CARE AND ATTENTION, YOU NEED TO
KNOW WHAT A BLESSING YOUR WRITING IS TO THOSE OF US
RECEIVING IT. YOUR TENDER, HONEST WORDS REMIND US ALL OF THE
DAILY GIFTS WE TAKE FOR GRANTED. THEY HAVE URGED ME TO STOP
AND NOTICE THE LOVE AND BEAUTY ALL AROUND ME IN WAYS I
OFTEN DON'T DUE TO THE BUSYNESS. THAT BUSYNESS, I MUST

REALIZE, IS MY CHOICE. THEREFORE, I CAN—AND I MUST—CHOOSE MORE WISELY. THANK YOU FOR THE LESSON.

YOUR WORDS ALSO DEMYSTIFY FOR US WHAT IT'S LIKE TO SIT WITH A FRIGHTENING DISEASE. BY PULLING BACK THE VEIL, YOU MAKE US ALL LESS AFRAID. YOUR COURAGE AND PEACE ARE REMARK-ABLE. THEY GIVE US ALL STRENGTH.

GOD BLESS YOU AND HEAL YOU. I KEEP YOU IN MY THOUGHTS AND PRAYERS DAILY. PRAYER WORKS.

Dr. Roy, whose wife forwarded my e-mail to him, writes:

KAYE SENT YOUR E-MAIL TO ME. HOW MEANINGFUL. YOU WRITE BEAUTIFULLY. YOUR FOCUS IS WHAT I WOULD HOPE FOR ALL OF MY PATIENTS AND WHAT I WOULD HOPE FOR MYSELF. THE SPIRITUAL JOURNEY YOU ARE BEGINNING IS SO VERY MOVING TO WITNESS. THE FREEDOM YOU HAVE GIVEN YOURSELF TO EXPERIENCE GOD'S LOVE AND GRACE WILL STRENGTHEN YOU FOREVER. I HAVE ALWAYS BEEN SURPRISED HOW HEALING THE TEARS ARE. I NOW CRY FOR YOU AND JIM FOR YOUR SUFFERING AND YOUR FREEDOM. I HAVE NOT TRIED TO FORCE MYSELF ON YOU IN YOUR EARLY STAGES OF ALL THIS. IT WOULD BE AN HONOR FOR ME TO SIT WITH YOU ALL EITHER IN QUIET OR JUST A VISIT. I WANT TO DO THIS BUT I DO NOT WANT TO INTRUDE. KEEP SITTING. LOVE TO YOU BOTH.

WOULD YOU MIND IF I SHARED YOUR NOTE WITH OTHERS WHO WORK WITH PATIENTS WITH LIFE-THREATENING ILLNESSES?

Roy has a gift with elderly people. He is Grandpa's doctor as well as the rest of our family. I watched his proactive ways of dealing with death as he cared for some of the people we love who are now gone—my parents, Jim's mother—but to think that what I write can be of value to people I don't know is exciting. What is happening with these e-mails and the messages passed out to cyberspace?

I have been working on writing for the past ten years. I even put out tentative stabs at publication, but never with perseverance. Just as with my spiritual practices, I now feel as if an apprenticeship is being launched into another sphere.

My e-mail team is turning into an intimate connection. I find this quote from Hauerwas's *Naming the Silence* in my journal, "When we or someone we love is suffering, what we need is not an explanation of the suffering, but a community of persons who will stand with us and help us absorb that suffering." My church family, our family, and close friends are such a community, but the growing e-mail group expands the community into a magical source of healing.

I am intrigued by the spontaneity permeating the e-mail responses. A handwritten note, executed with a more deliberate hand, has a more studied tone. Somehow, early in the morning perhaps, words flow from the fingers at the keyboard with the ease of a conversation in a rocking chair on the front porches we no longer occupy.

As I struggle with my own understanding of God, I treasure the affirmation that others are asking the same questions. My current obsession with the meaning of prayer—admitting out loud or in print of an attempt to communicate with God—feels as if I am treading on risky territory. At the beginning, even writing these words made me nervous. Shouldn't you graduate from divinity school before talking about this stuff? My confrontation with death opens a heavy, locked door. But once I ask the questions out loud or write about prayer in my e-mails, I realize many pilgrims are on this road, are seeking the quest, and welcome the dialogue.

Chemo Three

I have my third chemo on June 23, the third day of summer. My world centers on a day of chemo every third Friday. My blood pressure is down, 127 over 69. It goes down slightly more with each chemo round. The nurses are familiar. Michele is again in charge of my day of drugs.

I now know that I don't need to arrive at the suggested hour of 7:30, as I'll just sit in the waiting room for half an hour, so I get there at 7:55 and go right in. Michele accesses my port with the inch-and-a-half-long needle that I can look at for the first time. She draws blood and sends it up to the lab and the usual drill of analysis, prescription writing, and waiting for meds begins. The nurse comes in each session to say they are unusually slow that day and are still waiting for the written orders from my doctor. Each time, the process that should take an hour takes two. I wait in my little ten-by-fourteen foot cubical in my blue Barcalounger, wrapped in a cotton blanket heated up in the nifty blanket microwave. Wonderful friends are divided into three shifts. In a pattern consistent with chemo one and two, they start the meds at 10:00 AM Carole H. is keeping me company again today. I have brought the first twenty pages of my journal, which I have typed out and begin to think of as a book rather than just a journal. Carole reads it to me out loud. It sounds so different coming from another voice. She is an excellent editor and gives great suggestions for a change of verb here, pronoun there. She teaches Latin at a private, girls' high school and explains the use of the "historical present." Switching from past to present tense is a standard practice in Latin literature to bring immediacy to the scene. My story may not be up there with Caesar's campaigns, but it is central to my life. Carole's encouraging words edge me forward in my writing.

Jim comes at lunch time to see how I'm doing and to bring sustenance. He was at Vanderbilt earlier this morning as well. Jim's last PSA test has regrettably shown the prostate cancer is not contained, and he is undergoing six weeks of radiation. He goes to Vanderbilt early each morning, Monday through Friday, on his way to work, for a fifteen-minute zap of radiation. He is physically so strong that the treatment seems to have little effect on his stamina. The double-dipping, the husband/wife zapping, seems surreal.

When Jim leaves, I am still doing OK. Coping with chemo means finding distractions: I focus on my book, but I find another distraction as well. Ellen and I have been plotting for the last month over the phone about the possibility of chemo in Spain. I am determined to spend the entire month of August on my beloved island of Mallorca, at our magical beach house rented each summer, five yards from the Mediterranean Sea. Leaving Nashville later or coming home early for chemo five is an option I choose not to take. CHOP+R is a common treatment. There is an excellent hospital in Mallorca. Through my brother's contacts in Madrid, I have already accessed the number for the oncology department at the hospital in the capital city of Palma and the name of the doctor. I have called. They are familiar with CHOP+R. After the second call, they remember the American lady calling from Tennessee, and I have already set up an appointment for the procedure on the appropriate third Friday, August 5, thank you very much. Some of my friends are horrified. Don't they think Spanish people get sick? Daddy spent a month in this hospital on his last trip to Spain. I have not spoken to Dr. Greer because he has been on vacation, and I suspect he has not spent sufficient time in Europe to be comfortable with the idea of chemo abroad. But I'll deal with that issue when he returns. Today, I want to find out everything I can about the insurance issues of a treatment in a foreign country.

The chemo nurse, Michele, has agreed to call the manager of physician billing, Jody Rowland, so I can speak with her. She turns out to be an enthusiastic lady whom the hospital recruited from another city for her special skills. Health-care billing is more difficult, I suspect, than learning Chinese. She comes in to talk to me while I am in my chair with the drip. How accommodating is that? She catches on to my quest, seems delighted to have a challenge, and goes off to see what she can find out about BlueCross BlueShield benefits from the other side of the puddle. She comes back to my chemo cubical later in the afternoon with only two oncologists listed as BCBS providers in any of the information she found. They are both in Madrid. We could always fly to Madrid for the day, but I hope this will be a last-resort option.

I hope I'll finish early today. The Rituxan can be administered more quickly as I have shown no ill effects from previous chemos. Every few hours, I unplug the rolling IV pole and walk around the semi-circle of chemo cubicles to the ladies room to pee. After the Adriamycin, which I'm glad I didn't know is called the "red devil" until after the fourth round of treatment, my pee is pink. At two, they come in and tell me my magnesium count is low, and they have to give me a supplement through another drip. It can't be mixed with the CHOP+R meds, so I get another needle in my left arm and another bag on my left side. This drip will take two hours. Two hours!

Why couldn't they have started earlier? There goes my early departure. Decisions about treatments go through so many chains of command that efficiency takes a backseat to precaution. I could get into an agitated state. I could be really pissed. Or I could relax and accept the fact that the day will be long. My choice. Pick one. I'm not enduring the additional medical mix alone. My friends provide ongoing companionship. When I do finish, I'm fifteen minutes from home, my cozy bed, and my lush garden, and I don't have to report to an office the next day. I think I'll pick door number two, stay calm. The day goes slowly by as the meds drip into my system, and as usual I feel mild nausea, fatigue, and flu-like symptoms, especially during the last half hour when the bag of Rituxan is dripping at the highest dose of 400 ccs. I have been told that each chemo will be slightly more debilitating, but I have not found this true for me.

As strange liquids drip into both sides of my body, I remember that each day we choose whether our glass is half-empty or half-full and then live with the consequences of the view we choose. I watch people who travel overreact to delays and luggage losses. I want to say, "Stay home." If you travel, you are going to deal with all these issues at some point. The odds are inevitable. My parents, who traveled all the time, chose "rage mode." I watched for years as they quarreled and fretted between departure and arrival, and I decided I didn't need to follow that path. I am always grateful for the gift they gave me. By accompanying them on so many trips, I feel comfortable and at home in many parts of the globe and am fairly competent in a couple of foreign languages. But I have learned to leave out the rage over imperfect plans. I have learned to stay calm during travel's inevitable glitches. The practice helps me now dealing with the constant inconveniences and blunders associated with cancer. At this moment, I realize I have a choice. So I work on some deep breathing during the last two hours of plastic bags emptying into my veins.

When I go to the bathroom for the fifth time before leaving the hospital, I look down and see I have wet myself. Gross. Loss of control increases with each chemo and is my *worst* side effect. Another deep breath and I put my purse over my lower body and walk to the car with as much dignity as I can find. Maybe nausea would have been better. Maybe this is nausea. While we're discussing down there, I might as well tell you that most of that hair is gone, as well as the hair on my arms and legs. I still have half my eyebrows and lashes, so I lucked out. One friend confessed to losing every blade of hair, and when she stepped out of the tub and glimpsed herself in the mirror she thought she was an alien from the film *Close Encounters*. I also can go to the store and buy Kotex instead of Depends. A sixty-year-old woman buying . . . oh, never mind.

When I get home, I take a long, cleansing shower and notice the bug bites are completely gone, again. I take it as a good sign and go sit on my side porch to add summer garden air to my ribcage cavity. June is not the best garden month in Nashville. Spring perennials have blossomed out and later summer flowers—hollyhocks, cleome, and the flowering bushes of buddleia, rose of Sharon, and crepe myrtle—are yet to shine. Experimenting over the years with additional annuals to fill the gap has often been disappointing, as they look worse and worse as the heat intensifies. I have switched to leaves and grasses. I love the rich purple and jazzy chartreuse of the sweet potato vine (leaves), the wide range of leaf colors offered in the *Coleus* family and red grasses with delicate, pink, feathery plumes, the silver foliage of lamb's ear and the new foot-wide leaves of the butterbur plant, the citrus-yellow barberry bush, the fountain-shaped cardoon and the purple acanthus and pineapple lily. As I mature as a gardener, varying texture is more exciting than a new rose. Throw in a few pink-wave petunias for a flower touch and the combination continues to thrive until the first frost, and the new-wave petunias stay full with no deadheading necessary.

Mind on Mallorca

⟨ornament⟩

The remaining days of June and the beginning of July roll by slowly with little on the agenda. My bridge group usually adjourns for the summer, but because of my illness everyone makes a supreme effort to continue to play throughout the month of July. We never talk about this change in routine. They just continue to clear their calendars and show up. We play each Tuesday at our house, and I look forward to the therapy as much as the cards. My only other diversion is preparing for my big August birthday bash in Mallorca.

Back during the winter, before my diagnosis, I invited eighteen couples to our house for drinks in hopes of enticing them to come to Mallorca for my birthday. Peggy, the youngest member of the group and whose friendship blossomed in the volunteer trenches, brought Spanish cheeses to munch as I handed out information on the island and the hotels. Fifteen couples committed to the trip to Spain. I also invited a couple from London and another from Paris to round out the number to thirty-four. Counting Jim and me, my brother, Kevin, his wife, Barbara, and Nicky, whose husband Bill could not physically make the trip, we would have thirty-nine revelers for a week in Mallorca.

I invited Carole and John, Dana and Tom, and Nicky to stay at our house, the girls coming a week early to help with the plans. They had been at the scene two summers before when the idea of the party was born, which was the criterion to decide who would stay with us. The downside for them was sharing a bath and having no air conditioning.

I had perfect spots for the rest of the guests—two "hotel interiors," the name for family homes that have been restored and turned into small boutique hotels. One, Hotel San Jaume, is in Alcúdia, next to the Museum House where I grew up. It is still family owned, run by the grandson and his German wife, and rooms run about 100 euros a night. I remember as a child I could see the blue and white tile patio by bending out a third-floor window of the Museum House.

The other choice, about three miles away, is on the road between Alcúdia and the Port of Pollença, a spectacular house on a hill. Hotel Llenaire is coincidentally run by the grandchildren of the original owners as well, Michael and his brother-in-law Alex. The price tag for the sweeping view across Port of Pollença Bay from the swimming pool patio is 300 euros a night. I am delighted to offer two unique choices and price options.

Everyone is invited to come a few days early or stay a few days late with official, scheduled plans and activities arranged for the group from Wednesday, August 17 through Saturday night, August 20, the night of the big birthday bash. Another dozen friends who live or spend summers on the island are invited for Saturday night. The excitement of sharing my island with my own mob keeps me going!

Next Stop: The Mountains

∽

At the end of the month of June, I switch gears again and drive Grandpa Jim to his house on Monteagle Mountain for an extended Fourth of July weekend. With each of the chemo treatments, I should be feeling weaker, but I have not experienced this symptom and the hour-and-twenty-minute drive to the mountains is relatively easy. We usually go to Ponte Vedra for the Fourth, but since Jim's dad can no longer drive up to his mountain home by himself and the summers he has left to enjoy his favorite spot are dwindling, Jim, Jamie, Lisa, and I decide to share the weekend with him in Monteagle—with the babies, of course.

When we arrive, the temperature is ten degrees cooler than Nashville. It has been so hot at home for the last few weeks that I haven't been exercising, but here my feet are itching to walk. Grandpa's house is one of about 160 cottages that make up the Monteagle Sunday School Assembly. Founded in the 1880s, Monteagle was originally based on the Chautauqua system, retreat centers for families to gather in the summertime with educational and recreational activities. The assembly was one of many retreats people founded in the 1800s to go to higher ground and cooler temperatures to avoid summer heat and malaria. Grandpa courted his wife, Anne, while spending summertime on the mountain when they were both in their twenties. They bought a place of their own about thirty-five years ago. They would move to the mountain from May through September when Grandma was still alive. Grandpa chaired the Assembly board and retains involvement in the community. Grandpa, sitting on his front porch in his wicker rocker, smoking his pipe and reading his book, is a fixture in Monteagle summer life. Artist Anne Brothers's watercolor of the scene hangs in the cottage to officially preserve the memory.

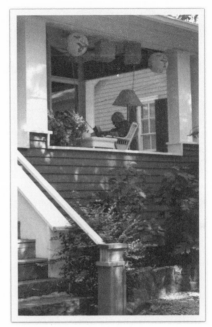

Grandpa on the porch at Monteagle.

Grandpa's Victorian cottage was built in 1890. The house, navy-blue clapboard with white trim and white wicker porch furniture, provides a perfect setting for flags and watermelon and apple pie and the passing Fourth of July parade of decorated tricycles and bikes and hundreds of children in variations of red, white, and blue t-shirts and shorts and sundresses.

Grandpa talked about selling the Monteagle house. The roof leaks. There is no real shower. The kitchen has a mildewed, old fridge and nasty linoleum peeling up from the floor. At eighty-seven, my father-in-law finds the repairs daunting.

My own dad lived to be eighty-six. He knew in the spring of that last year he could no longer travel to Spain in June. His summer routine of his excavation in Mallorca had never been broken. He died in May. I remember Dr. Roy's sensitivity to the importance of what an elderly person has to look forward to, and I knew that we couldn't let Grandpa sell his Monteagle cottage. We all talked over the course of the weekend and decided to renovate, starting with a tin roof and a real shower.

My favorite part about Grandpa's cottage is the front bedroom upstairs. The walls and peaked ceiling are the original pine tongue-and-groove wood, the floors wide-plank pine. I open the side window and front door to a second-floor porch, lie on the bed, and let the cross breeze flow over my feet. At home I would be a prisoner of air conditioning. Here I enjoy the moderate afternoon breeze, read my book until I fall asleep. This treetop room is a haven for the extra naps I need. At night I again sleep soundly and wake up first to the sound of crickets, and slightly later, bird songs. One always follows behind the other, as if taking their turn. There seem to be more birds here than in Nashville, but perhaps it is the huge tree that reaches above my second-floor window.

Grandpa and I spend two quiet days, mostly on the porch, before the rest of the family arrives. These moments on the porch, like moments in my garden, expand with accelerated meaning as I relish the space, the cool air, the hosta leaves in the bed across the street. The little things. Grandpa is bent over with an osteoporotic arch, but he is still here with us, the last member of his generation in our family. Facing my own mortality, I see him in a new light as he reads and I type. People passing by come and visit to catch up with Grandpa, tell him he is missed when he is not in his chair on the porch. The rest of the family arrives on Saturday. The rustic charm of the porch is immediately transformed by an invasion of plastic: plastic baby swing, plastic baby carrier, plastic tricycle, assorted dump trucks. Grandpa is the only familiar fixture in his chair, reading his latest science-fiction book, with the rickety, brass lamp held together with grey duct tape.

The first night, we have dinner with Nicky and Bill and their children and grandchildren in their mountain house just outside the Assembly grounds. We eat outside on one of the wide porches, overlooking the valley down towards Nashville. Our children set off fireworks for their children, whose wide-eyed delight is the highlight of the show.

At noon on the next day, the communal picnic is set up in the large, green common in the middle of the Assembly grounds, dominated by a Victorian gazebo complete with an old-time band. Imagine makeshift tables of six-foot-by-thirty-inch pieces of plywood each supported by two sawhorses. Imagine as many tables as could possibly fit on an acre of lawn while leaving just enough space for the folding wood-slat chairs and for people to maneuver sideways in-between. Add a slight slant to all the wood tops that are stored for the rest of the year in a space without temperature control. A family name on duct

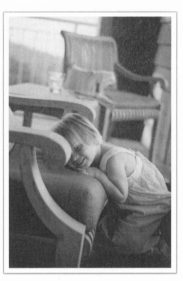

Granddaugher Baker flirting.

tape identifies each board. The allotted spot for each family is sacred. In the morning, each family covers their table with their own version of a red, white, and blue cloth and patriotic centerpieces. Wooden figures of Uncle Sam from one of the mountain craft shops and baskets of wildflowers, many with a few flags, add color to the setting. Right before the picnic begins, family members arrive carrying abundant platters of fried chicken, barbecue, cut fruit in carved-out watermelons, and every flavor of cake. After watching the children's parade, all ages cram together to feast, catch up, be interviewed and interrogated by the older generation, and checked out by the younger generation.

I sit with an old friend, Martha, from Junior League volunteer days, whom I had seen with a head scarf in Dr. Greer's office on an early visit and hadn't had a chance to hear her whole story. Today her scarf is an American flag pattern. Wigs are just too hot for the summer; so much for my major investment. She explains that she has non-Hodgkin's lymphoma and has also been treated with CHOP+R. The tumor in her stomach shrank but is still there, and she is scheduled for a stem-cell transplant in the fall. I remember on an early visit Dr. Greer listing a stem-cell transplant as one of my options down the road should the cancer return. Martha can use her own stem cells. I wouldn't have that option as my systemic disease has contaminated all of my cells. My best bet will be a match with my only sibling, my brother in Spain. Kevin would go to a lab and have blood drawn, and then, Dr. Greer pointed out, would come the tricky part. The blood would have to be transported back to Nashville to be tested. I have already talked to my brother. He reassures me, "This will not be a problem. One of our closest friends has a company that ships blood, plasma, etc., all over the world in temperature-controlled containers." The workable plan, ready to go, is left for the moment on the back burner and I will add Martha to my prayer list.

The rest of July passes as I return to my routine in Nashville. I continue the meetings once a week with Ken, bridge on Tuesdays, and preparations for Mallorca. Carole helps me with a smashing invitation, printed on her computer, for the Saturday birthday dinner in Mallorca. I find some Crane stationery, heavy cards with wavy lines of aqua and orange that remind me of the rhythm of the water going down the left side and the same pattern lining the envelopes. Carole uses an aqua ink and contemporary font from her software program, and you would never know the invitations are not professionally printed. Both detail queens are thrilled. I type a tentative schedule of events: where we will go for dinner, who is invited to our house each day for lunch by the sea. I even find funny place cards, one set with fish and one set with boats to use for two of the dinners. The most important items ready to be put in my suitcase are sixteen sets of watercolors, brushes, pens, and watercolor paper. I have warned the invitees that my birthday present request is something put on a four-by-six inch piece of watercolor paper, a painting or a poem or whatever their imagination dictates.

Dr. Greer returns from a family vacation in France, and I call to talk about the possibility of August's chemo in Mallorca. The July chemo, the fourth chemo in the middle of this month, is the benchmark. I will go two weeks after this treatment for another PET scan to determine the status of the Richter's cancer. It is hoped, it will be gone. If any cancer remains, I will have four more treatments. If I am cancer free, I will have two more treatments, six total. The chemo in Mallorca will be number five. The protocol for treatment is to automatically perform two extra, precautionary treatments, even if no cancer remains, to help prevent recurrences. The downside of extra treatments, in my case, is that the CHOP+R is so strong that it can only be administered a certain number of times to one person. In my case, the doctor "guestimates," about ten in all.

I can tell Dr. Greer is skeptical about medicine in Mallorca, but is being a good sport dealing with a stubborn woman. I have not met with Dr. Greer since before the first chemo. Jim meets with his doctor each week during his six weeks of radiation. When I ask Dr. Greer's nurse, Ellen, if no scheduled meeting is unusual, she explains that I didn't have any problems that required a meeting with him. On the phone today, he brings up the money issue and the possibility of insurance not covering the cost abroad. He asks if I realize the cost of the Rituxan. I tell him I just know our bill reflects a cost of about $3,000 per chemo treatment, all but a few hundred dollars covered by insurance. He says the Rituxan costs $25,000 per treatment. "You mean $2,500?" "No, $25,000." The drug companies are out of control. Each chemo bill we receive starts out at $10,000 to $12,000, sometimes more. The hospital negotiates with the insurance company and they settle on a much lower figure such as the $3,000. But for people who have no insurance, there is no negotiation. The most destitute patient just gets the original bill, which, of course, they cannot pay. The system is ridiculous, outrageous, nuts.

I also ask Dr. Greer how he feels about the upcoming PET scan results. "Oh, I'm sure you will have good test results. I'm sure that the cancer is gone." "Wow. How can you be so sure?" "It will be gone." Then he pauses as if weighing whether to say more. "But that doesn't mean it's not coming back." A gift is given and taken away in the same breath. "What do you mean?" "Well, you knew that." "I did?" I hadn't given one thought to the situation beyond the pronounce-ment of the Richter's cure. The cancer was coming back? I hadn't given one breath to the consequences of my "chronic" CLL and the strong likelihood of another cancer appearing in one of my unsus-pecting and vulnerable lymph nodes. I didn't want to think about my world after this round, not yet. But the seed is planted and now taking root in the back of my brain.

I call one of my cancer-survivor friends, Sally, after the conversation. "Don't worry, the doctor gives you the worst-case scenario, and there is always a chance that a cancer will recur. But think of all the people you know, like me, who have survived breast cancer for decades."

I call Dr. Greer's nurse, Ellen, and she is out of the office for a week's vacation. When she is back, I call again.

"Why is Dr. Greer so certain the Richter's is gone?"

"I have never seen a patient undergo that strong a chemo and sail through with such ease. You are the new poster child. You were able to tolerate the full dosages on schedule. You will have a good report."

Ellen dodges the question about recurrences. I joke with her about deserting me, about not being in the office when Dr. Greer returned, and I tell her the details of my conversation trying to convince him a chemo in Spain will be OK. I need her on my team. She laughs. "I should have given you my home number. I was there. We used to go to the beach for spring break, but I just couldn't swing it this year." I knew she was a single mom with two teenage kids, and money was probably tight. I wanted her kids to have that week at the beach. Maybe I could open a door.

Chemo Four

*T*omorrow is July 14, the date for chemo four. In another two weeks I will have the second PET scan to determine my cancer status. Dr. Roy has felt under both arms and thinks it's gone. I hope so. I go in a day early and give Ellen the keys to our place in Ponte Vedra, pressing them into her hand. "You and your kids are going to Florida for another week's vacation, not subject to negotiation." I see some tears. Jim and I don't share our Florida home, but this woman has just become the exception to the rule. End of discussion. When I tell Jim, he totally agrees. OK, I actually told him after the fact, but I have learned over the years that it's easier to seek forgiveness than permission.

By the fourth chemo, I am an old hand with the drugs, the order in which they will be administered, the time each will take, the effects each will have. As I look back, my consciousness of what was happening to me during the first chemo was about 30 percent, rising to about 50 percent with the second chemo, slightly higher on the third. Only with the fourth chemo is my mind completely engaged with each step. Only with the fourth chemo is all the information, all the procedures, all the lethal drugs dripping into my body, hour after hour, fully registering in my mind.

My day of chemo four goes smoothly—from the anti-nausea drug Zofran through the CHOP+R and to the flush with a 500 mg bag of saline, 5 ccs of heparin saline, and finally a third saline flush of

10 ccs—then I'm unhooked and ready to go home. Flushing the port to keep it free of infection is always part of the drill.

While I am in my Barcalounger with drip I have found out Rituxan is called Magma Thera in Europe. The next day I call Ellen and ask her to put in writing the exact meds for my treatment so they can be faxed to the hospital in Mallorca and they can then send me an estimate of the cost. E-mail is not on their radar. Maybe they are not as sophisticated as I thought. I am extremely concerned about the insurance issues and the cost, although I know European prices will be considerably less. Then I have a brain flash. On one of the sheets Jody gave me is a number for international inquiries for BlueCross BlueShield. I call. After a reasonable wait, I speak with a woman who informs me that my BlueCross BlueShield coverage will be honored at any accredited hospital in Europe using the same procedures as in the U.S. I don't need to worry about paying ahead, about the price for Rituxan, about flying to Madrid. Yippee.

The day before chemo, I compose another e-mail message:

UPDATE FROM PATIENT SIGGY
JULY 14, 2005
DEAR FRIENDS,

TOMORROW IS CHEMO FOUR. NUMBER FOUR IS THE TURNING POINT BECAUSE TWO WEEKS AFTER NUMBER FOUR, I WILL HAVE A SECOND PET SCAN. I'LL GO INTO THE VANDY RADIOLOGY LAB AND SIT QUIETLY WHILE A NICE TECHNICIAN REMOVES SOME OF MY BLOOD. ANOTHER TECHNICIAN IN A NEARBY LAB WILL INJECT THE RETRACTED BLOOD WITH RADIOACTIVE MATERIAL. NO, THIS IS NOT A SCIENCE-FICTION MOVIE. THE FIRST TECHNICIAN WILL MANIPU-LATE THE BLOOD BACK INTO MY ARTERIES AND PUT ME IN ONE OF THOSE STREAMLINED METAL MACHINES WHERE OTHER TECHNICIANS WITH ADDITIONAL TRAINING WILL OBSERVE THE NEW FLOW. GOOD NEWS, I AM NOT CLAUSTROPHOBIC.

THIS SPECIAL TEST IS RESERVED FOR CANCER PATIENTS. THE RADIOACTIVE STUFF PICKS UP ANY PLACES IN MY BODY WHERE BIG,

BAD CELLS ARE LURKING. IN THE PET SCAN, BEFORE THE FIRST CHEMO, THE ONLY BIG CELLS WERE UNDER BOTH ARMS. THE BEST-CASE SCENARIO, AFTER THIS SCAN, WILL BE THAT THE BAD CANCER CELLS HAVE COMPLETELY DISAPPEARED. IF THAT IS THE CASE, I WILL ONLY HAVE TWO MORE CHEMOS. IF THERE IS STILL SOME CANCER, THEY WILL DO FOUR MORE CHEMOS.

PLEASE BRING OUT THE PRAYER MATS.

NOW, YOU WANT TO KNOW SOMETHING SCARY? THE ORIGINAL MEDICAL PLAN DID NOT INCLUDE A PRE-CHEMO PET SCAN. MY THEORY IS THAT THE CALL FOR A PET SCAN BEFORE CHEMO NUMBER ONE HAD JUST SLIPPED BETWEEN THE CRACKS. TOO MANY DETAILS WITH TOO MANY PATIENTS; I WAS LUCKY TO BE WORKED IN QUICKLY. ONE OF MY OTHER SPECIAL DOCTOR FRIENDS MENTIONED THE ADVANTAGE OF A PET SCAN, AND WHEN JIM AND I MET WITH DR. GREER BEFORE THE FIRST CHEMO, I MENTIONED THE POSSI-BILITY AND DR. GREER SCHEDULED THE PROCEDURE. THE FIRST SCAN WILL BE A BENCHMARK MEASURE FOR THE SECOND. THE WHOLE PATIENT EXPERIENCE AT VANDERBILT HAS BEEN VERY POSI-TIVE, BUT VANDY IS A LARGE MEDICAL CENTER WITH HUNDREDS OF DOCTORS, PATIENTS, AND STUDENT DOCTORS. YOU ABSOLUTELY NEED TO BE YOUR OWN ADVOCATE, ALL THE TIME, EVERY DAY. THE TWO PET SCANS WILL BE MAJOR, IN MY VIEW.

NOW, AN UPDATE. FOR THOSE OF YOU WHO WERE PAYING ATTENTION, YOU WILL REMEMBER THAT I HAVE TWO CANCERS, OR ACTUALLY TWO VERSIONS OF THE SAME CANCER. I HAVE CLL, CHRONIC LYMPHOCYTIC LEUKEMIA, WHICH IS A SLOW-GROWING, MILD CANCER THAT SOME PEOPLE HAVE FOR MANY YEARS WITH LITTLE EFFECT OTHER THAN FATIGUE AND SUSCEPTIBILITY TO FEVERS AND FLUS. AS ONE DOCTOR FRIEND TOLD ME, IF YOU HAVE TO HAVE CANCER, THIS IS THE ONE TO PICK. FIVE PERCENT OF THE PEOPLE WITH CLL HAVE A TRANSFORMATION TO A MORE RAPIDLY PROGRESSIVE LYMPHOMA. I AM ONE OF THE LUCKY FIVE PERCENT, AND THESE TRANSFORMED, NASTY LITTLE DEVILS ARE WHAT WE ARE TARGETING WITH THE AGGRESSIVE AND POTENT CHEMO CALLED CHOP+R.

ACCORDING TO THE CANCER GRAPEVINE, I AM SUPPOSED TO BECOME MORE FATIGUED, FEEL SICKER WITH EACH CHEMO, BUT MY BODY DIDN'T GET THE MESSAGE AND I HAVE BEEN DOING GREAT. THE REASON THAT YOU HAVEN'T HEARD FROM ME FOR A WHILE IS:

ONE: I HAVE BEEN OVERWHELMED WITH THE POWERFUL RESPONSES TO MY E-MAILS. THE FEEDBACK FROM SO MANY OF YOU IS LIKE A HEALING DRUG. I SPEND SIGNIFICANT TIME RESPONDING TO EVER-INCREASING, MUCH-APPRECIATED E-MAILS. SOMETHING MAGICAL IS HAPPENING. PLEASE KEEP THE RESPONSES COMING; YOU MIGHT BE IN MY BOOK.

MY NEAR-DEATH EXPERIENCE WITH MY DIAGNOSIS AND THOUGHTS OF THE WORST-CASE SCENARIO FROM RICHTER'S SYNDROME (THAT'S ANOTHER WORD FOR THE TRANSFORMATION) IS COUNTERACTED BY THE POWER OF THOUSANDS OF PRAYERS THAT SURROUND ME ALL THE TIME AND GIVE ME A SERENE INNER PEACE AND THE KNOWLEDGE THAT SO MANY DEAR FRIENDS CARE ABOUT ME, ARE THINKING OF ME.

REMEMBER THE WOMAN ABOUT WHOM I WROTE WHO FELT DIMINISHED BY CANCER, WHO THOUGHT HER FRIENDS AND COLLEAGUES COULDN'T DEAL WITH HER DISEASE AND TURNED AWAY AND MADE HER FEEL INVISIBLE? I CAN'T HELP CONTINUING TO THINK ABOUT HER. I HAVE HAD THE OPPOSITE EXPERIENCE. I AM ENLARGED, STANDING ON A TABLE IN THE MIDDLE OF A STAGE, SURROUNDED BY APPLAUSE. THE APPLAUSE COMES FROM MY TEAM. I STARTED WITH A CONTACT LIST OF EIGHTEEN. NOW OUR TEAM IS OVER ONE HUNDRED. THANK YOU IS INSUFFICIENT.

TWO: I HAVE BEEN WRITING A BOOK ABOUT MY EXPERIENCE. I KNOW, TOO MANY PEOPLE GO THROUGH A CRISIS AND WANT TO WRITE ABOUT IT. WELL, IT'S YOUR FAULT. YOU'VE ENCOURAGED MY WRITING. I CAN'T STOP.

THE STORY STARTS WITH DAY ONE, WHEN A ROUTINE VISIT TO OUR INTERNIST, ROY, FOR AN ANTIBIOTIC FOR AN ALLERGIC REACTION TO BUG BITES, TURNED INTO A FULL DAY AT VANDERBILT AND A DIAGNOSIS THAT NIGHT OF B-CELL LYMPHOMA. FOUR DAYS LATER, THE DIAGNOSIS CHANGED TO CLL AND TWO DAYS AFTER THAT RICHTER'S TRANSFOR-MATION WAS ADDED TO THE MIX. I'M CONFUSED TOO.

HAIR UPDATE

I STILL HAVE SOME EYEBROWS AND LASHES. MORE CANCER GRAPEVINE REVEALS THAT SOME PEOPLE LOSE THEM AND SOME DON'T. THE GRAPEVINE IS KEY. I ASKED THE NURSE IN ONCOLOGY IF PEOPLE LOST THEM AND SHE DIDN'T KNOW. I ALSO HAVE A SMALL PATCH OF HAIR ON THE TOP OF MY HEAD THAT WOULD STILL BE THERE IF IT HADN'T BEEN SHAVED OFF WHEN THE REST WAS GOING ANYWAY.

My expensive wig is too hot and too helmety and I've only worn it a few times. Connie has found some fabulous scarves on the Internet in a rainbow of colors. I love my scarves.

If I had refrained from shaving that small patch, I could have fashioned a modified mohawk or braided it like the last Emperor of China. Oops, I forgot. I'd already cut my hair short before it started to leave me. Scratch the last option.

Another no-hair perk: Rain was pouring down in massive quantities as I left the house to meet with my trainer, Janet, this morning. My damp scarf still looked perky as I entered the exercise room and it added a refreshing touch to the workout.

Guess where chemo five will be? At the hospital on the Island of Mallorca, not far from the magical house by the sea where we will spend the rest of the month. So is chemo slowing me down? I don't think so.

I continue to feel the power of your love surrounding me, and I know I am healing.

Hugs, Sigourney

Within a day my inbox is crowded with uplifting responses full of hugs and prayers and thoughts and thanks.

Barbara C. writes:

I think we are the ones benefiting from your e-mails.

And my brother, who is not religious, writes:

However, I am totally convinced of the power of positive thinking and its effects on healing, especially when multiplied by the effects of many people thinking positively about the same cause at the same time. Therefore, I am one of the many (there are many more than one hundred) who is standing there applauding and cheering you on to victory. Go for it, baby! Kick ass, honey! Boo to the bad cancer cells.

Patricia, writes that her husband, David, a rabbi:

WOULD GO TO THE SYNAGOGUE TODAY AND SAY SPECIAL PRAYERS BY THE TORAH. HE TOLD ME THAT THE POWER OF PRAYER IS EXACTLY AS YOU DESCRIBE IT—SOMETHING THAT IS ALMOST TANGIBLE.

My friend Jane refers to my:

GROWING NUMBER OF PRAYER WARRIORS.

And Dorothy responds:

THE PATIENT HEALS HER FRIENDS.

Guna, a New York friend who knows very few of the rest of the e-mail team writes:

OFTEN FEEL AS IF ALL OF US ARE SITTING IN A CIRCLE HOLDING HANDS, LISTENING TO YOU, AND BEING WITH YOU.

Jan, one of my most loyal responders writes:

I TRY TO IMAGINE YOUR SCALP AND CANNOT QUITE GET THE PICTURE. YOUR SPIRIT, HOWEVER, IS ALMOST PALPABLE.

And even a college friend of Jamie's, whose last name is Campbell so they call him Soup, touches my heart when he writes:

. . . YOUR OVERWHELMING STRENGTH AND OPTIMISM JUST FLOW OUT OF YOUR MESSAGE.

I sit on my bed back home and look at the collection of yellow, plastic pill tubes with clumsy childproof tops on my dresser obscuring my collection of silvertopped crystal bottles clustered together in the back-right corner. I don't like plastic. I used to take two pills a day for hormones and blood pressure; now I take so many that it's hard to keep track. Maybe I should buy one of those partitioned boxes my father used to use to divide the pills into days of the week, another opportunity for plastic. I'm resisting. Each of these surrenders to age sends the message I won't always be around. Oh, one more symptom I forgot mention is numbness of the feet. It's a weird feeling, and I need to remember not to cross my ankles when I'm on the bed for afternoon naps and postdinner TV as that only makes the tingling worse.

Today is the nineteenth of July, my actual sixtieth birthday. The big celebration is moved to August because that is when we have the house in Mallorca. My bridge group comes for the day with a special celebratory lunch provided by Susie. After a long afternoon nap, Jim and I are invited to another birthday celebration at Nicky and Bill's with two other couples. I'm delighted to have the opportunity to have Bill as part of the celebration since he will not be able to come to Mallorca. So many places are not handicap accessible, and Bill has been confined to a wheelchair for years. His upbeat personality, optimistic spirit, and gift of engaging others in his causes for kids keep him going. On this particular evening, Nicky outdoes herself with Alaska king salmon cooked on the grill and a homemade, angel food cake with a boiled spun-sugar icing and strawberries.

Mountain High

*T*he next day I take Grandpa back up to his haven on Monteagle Mountain. I want to give him one more opportunity to sit on his porch before we take off for Mallorca. Jim's and my dances with cancer intensify the importance of quality time with the last member of the older generation in our family. I also want to talk to some other Monteagle friends about contractors and renovations and the tricks of navigating the notoriously rigid Assembly rules.

I anticipate a few more nights in my "tree-house" room with the morning cacophony of birds and crickets, but I'm dubious about dealing with the Assembly old guard. The closed ranks of this insular community can be jarring to any outsider and remind me of my early days in Nashville, thirty-eight years ago. I was so out of sync with the southern ways that are now so much a part of my heart.

I once heard someone remark, while referring to a couple who didn't fit the usual Assembly profile, "I wonder why they wanted to be up here anyway?" When I reported this comment to Grandpa, he said, in reference to the couple, "I don't know them." I wanted to say, "Grandpa, shame on you." It reminded me of Jim's maternal grand-mother who would listen to me talk about someone new I had met as a young bride in Nashville. She would lean forward and say, "Now, Dahlin'! Who are her people?"

It took me years to understand Southern talk. In the South, "I don't know Sue" really means "I want nothing to do with Sue."

"I would like to know Sue better" really means, "I'll be nice to Sue if I see her, but I have enough friends already and no extra time."

"She is so attractive, let's plan a dinner party and include Sue" means "I want to know Sue." It probably involves a friend you and Sue already have in common who has given you a call to tell you that Sue, one of her "best" friends, is moving to town.

In fairness to the Southern girl, she has kept up with her best friends from kindergarten and dozens of her sorority sisters from a large Southern college who settled in the same town. She has additional friends to keep up with through her husband's office and his former college fraternity. She has kids and carpools and has bonded with all those mothers who belonged to similar sororities at similar schools and who share evening potluck suppers. How many friends can one girl juggle?

I know for myself that if I didn't live in the South, I would never be surrounded by the multitude of friends whom I have made over many potluck suppers in our own backyard.

I spend time on the mountain catching up with more never-ending thank-you notes and working on my journal, which is definitely turning into a book. I work on the—OK, let's start calling it "book"—in the mornings, while my brain is fresh and my creative juices flow freely. My five-year-old laptop no longer holds any charge. The CD slot is broken, so the only way I can transfer files is with a flash drive, a nifty little gizmo about the size of a key ring that mysteriously holds hundreds of files. I don't have a printer but am told there is one in Winfield House, the woman's library, across the road from our cottage. I walk over three times before one of the computers is free. I insert the flash drive and try to print, but the printer is not working. I go back across the road to do my best without it, and now my flash drive will not work either. The teeth in the connector have been bent by the old printer in the library. When I arrive home, I decide on another expensive purchase—accelerated spending is clearly another symptom of my disease—and hit CompUSA for a new Sony VAIO laptop to take with me to Spain. It weighs less than three pounds and holds a charge for more than six hours because of the smaller screen. Happy birthday to me.

Benchmark PET Scan

O n July 27 I am back at Vanderbilt at 7:45 AM at the radiology department behind the main entrance to the hospital. I am relaxed, by myself, my blood pressure at 100 over 60, unbelievably low for a person who used to break into hives on entering the parking lot, let alone the hospital. Instead of just one test, this day I am scheduled to also have a MUGA scan to test for flow status of blood to the heart (strong chemo can screw that up), a chest x-ray for the chronic cough that has stayed with me since Memorial Day (another consequence of CLL), and most important, the PET scan to determine if all cancer cells have been zapped by the CHOP+R regime. When I arrive, they also inform me I am scheduled for a CAT scan, but what's another test? I think of the trauma most people experience who have to go for just one of these tests.

The MUGA scan lasts about an hour. The PET is longer because the nurse injects a radioactive sugar solution into my bloodstream, cold going in, and I wait for an hour while it circulates into my body. I sit in another blue naugahyde chair, trying to stay as still as possible. I drink the pink chalk shake and wait another half hour as the dye works into more hard-to-reach crevices. Then I can go through the machine.

The young nurse in charge of the PET scan room has long, beautiful red hair. I can't resist. "You have the most beautiful hair." "I'm losing it tomorrow," she replies. "I'm donating it to Locks of Love." She is giving her beautiful hair to a program for children with cancer. As I lie on the metal bed and my body moves in and out of the machine during half an hour of silence, I breathe in deeply and review not only the skill, but also the depth of caring of all of the people I encounter at Vanderbilt, from doctor to scheduler.

The next morning, Jim and I wait for Dr. Greer and the much-anticipated cancer status report. Jim checks his watch. Even with his daily radiation zaps, he is still on the tight time schedule I have left behind. Ellen peeks her head into our examination room and gives a thumbs up. I'm glad to hear the news from her, as she is the one I have been dealing with the most over the last three months.

When Dr. Greer comes in, he confirms the good news. The big cancer, the Richter's syndrome is gone, finito, history. I am elated. Dr. Greer hits me with another surprise. "You are doing so well, I really don't think a treatment in Mallorca will be necessary. Why ruin your vacation?"

"Really?" What a thought: just go and have a great time. "What about when I return? What about the other two? Do you think they are still necessary? Isn't there a certain logic in leaving well enough alone? After all, don't I need all the good cells possible to continue to fight the CLL?"

Dr. Greer responds, "We can continue to think about that. But let's schedule the next one after your return just in case."

"Explain to me more about what you said about the cancer coming back. Is the likelihood about the same as with breast cancer?"

"No. Because of the CLL there is a stronger chance of a recurrence. But it probably won't be Richter's. The CHQP+R has been very effective in eliminating that strain. It would be another, hopefully less-aggressive, cancer."

Focus on the present, not what might or might not happen in the future. I remember Ellen talking about why she loves working with hematology patients: so many of the diseases can be cured. I drive myself toward home on a high, full of energy. I pick up my cell phone to call someone with the good news, but it is out of juice. Another memory lapse; I forgot to recharge. I think of the missed opportunity as I navigate my special shortcuts out of Vanderbilt up by Love Circle, avoiding lights on the main artery. It is two o'clock by the time I come through the kitchen door. I eat half a sandwich, call the kids, call Grandpa, call key friends. I plan to meet Lisa later to shop for things for her house to fluff for the dinner party she is planning for Jamie's thirty-fifth birthday. I am so flattered she asked me to help shop. I want to celebrate a return to normal, but first an update. How great to send out the news to the ever-growing list, now at 150 people, by pressing a few buttons at the top of the inbox.

UPDATE FROM PATIENT SIGGY
JULY 28, 2005
DEAR FRIENDS,

I HAVE JUST COME FROM MY FOLLOW-UP MEETING WITH DR. GREER AND THE BIG, BAD RICHTER'S SYNDROME CANCER IS GONE, FINITO, TOAST. I THOUGHT NOTHING COULD BE BETTER NEWS UNTIL DR. GREER ALSO SAID THAT I WAS DOING SO WELL THAT HE THOUGHT I COULD SKIP THE JULY CHEMO IN MALLORCA AND JUST ENJOY THE MONTH HOLIDAY. HOW GREAT IS THAT? SO I AM OFF FOR AUGUST IN SPAIN TO THINK OF NOTHING BUT SUN AND SURF AND ENJOY OUR MAGICAL HOUSE BY THE SEA. I WILL SPEND A MONTH BEING A WELL PERSON WITHOUT HAVING TO THINK ABOUT DOCTOR'S OFFICES AND NEEDLES AND DRUGS BEING SIPHONED INTO MY VEINS.

I AM OFF TO FINISH PACKING SO THIS ONE HAS TO BE SHORT. I WILL GIVE DETAILS OF SPAIN WHEN I RETURN AT THE END OF THE MONTH.

HAVE A GREAT AUGUST.

HUGS, SIGOURNEY

I notice not all of the e-mails go successfully into e-mail land, but I am in too much of a hurry to figure out the glitch. I will worry about it later, and I do receive dozens of responses right away with so many exclamation points and "congratulations" that I feel as if the party has begun.

In fact, Linda writes:

YOU DESERVE TO BE ECSTATIC, AND LET'S GET THE PARTY STARTED. NOW ALL OF US HAVE MORE REASON TO CELEBRATE YOUR BIRTHDAY—YOU CONQUERING THAT BIG, BAD BUG IS A WONDERFUL GIFT TO ALL OF US.

Sandra claims that:

. . . WITH YOUR SENSE OF HUMOR YOU WILL STILL HAVE YOUR FOLLOWING . . . NOT TO WORRY, DEAR, PEOPLE LOVE A WARM HEART AND COUPLED WITH WIT AND GIGGLES, YOUR FOLLOWING WILL STILL BE WITH YOU.

And Ellen adds:

YOUR DESCRIPTIONS AND HEARTFELT INSIGHTS HAVE DONE SO MUCH TO INSPIRE US ALL AND I KNOW THEY WOULD BRING COMFORT TO SOMEONE GOING THROUGH AN EXPERIENCE SIMILAR TO YOURS.

A Month in Mallorca

$\mathcal{I}$am on vacation from cancer and the e-mail responses fuel my energy to work on my story and enjoy the month ahead. My less-than-three-pound Sony VAIO is in the side pocket of my carry-on. In three days I am off to Mallorca without the challenges of having chemo in Spain. I finish last-minute paperwork and instructions to my Nashville housecleaner and gardener. I review the piles of things on the dressing-room floor to go in my suitcases: fifteen t-shirts; ten pairs of capri pants; a couple pairs of shorts for walking (though I'm better in the extended coverage of capris); six shirts; four bathing suits with parea covers; four smashing new outfits for the birthday week; a dozen books; my journal; the watercolor sets and funny place cards with fish and boats for the dinners; my Revlon moisturizer; sunscreens; lipsticks; a couple of sticks and brushes for what remain of my eyebrows; pills; and toothpaste. A month is a long time.

I leave by myself for Mallorca on July 31. Jim can't come until August 4, but we have the house for the whole month and our middle son, Daniel, arrives tomorrow, August 1. I have an uneventful flight through Madrid and on to the fifth-largest airport in Europe, Palma de Mallorca. My luggage even makes it, always a 50–50 shot. I always pack a bathing suit and change of clothes in my carry-on just in case. I push the luggage through the parking lot to the bargain rental car arranged by my brother and take off on the familiar road across the island. The first half of the drive is a modern motorway to the center of the island and the industrial town of Inca, where leather goods are manu- factured. Once out of the city of Palma, I drive through the familiar farmland on both sides of the road, spotting stucco houses with wavy, red-tile roofs nestled into the hills along the way and field after field of almond and olive trees, clusters of sheep settled under scanty patches of shade, and a scattering of Don Quixote-like windmills, the former irrigation system. On the left are mountain ranges, Sierra de Alfabia and Sierra de Torellas, one flowing into the next, that follow me all forty miles across the northwestern side of the island ending at the tip of the Bay of Pollença. The 40-mile-square island has three large bays: the Palma Bay is at my back; the Bay of Pollença and the Bay of Alcúdia are on the other side of the island where I am headed. The latter two bays are right next to each other, separated only by a narrow finger of land. Our house is located on the left side of that finger, facing the Bay of Pollença.

On the other side of Inca, the road narrows to a rural road lined with dry-stack stone walls. As children, my brother and I would count off each small town we passed through—Santa Maria, Consell, Binisalem, Campanet—and know we were getting closer and closer to our destination, the town of Alcúdia. My spirits lift with each

familiar turn of the road and my mouth waters for the first taste of farm tomatoes, local Mahon cheese, and brown bread still hot from the oven. Just past Campanet, I take the cutoff for the town of Pollença, a

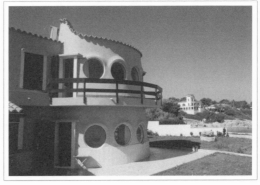

"El Barco."

detour to visit my brother for the first night. After a few miles, I circle the town and drive up into the valley of Son March. Kevin and Barbara bought the ruin of a stone farmhouse right after they were married, thirty-seven years ago, and have been turning it into paradise ever since, restoring and expanding with old doors and windows and Spanish antiques. The stone walls are the same color as the mountains. Even the kitchen sink is antique stone. I can still hear my father's voice saying, "Every inch of their house 'sings.'"

We sit out on the patio and have a light, Spanish lunch. After a year apart I am always struck by my brother's handsome, ageless face. A light sprinkle of grey in his thick, bark-brown hair is visible only at close range, with my glasses on. I sometimes wonder if a sorcerer is involved, and a Dorian Gray portrait with appropriate bags and sags is in the back of some closet. Barbara has more grey in her pale, sandy hair but she is a striking woman, reed-thin with regal bearing. We catch up on our grown children, their two boys, our three. Their younger son, Alexander, age thirty-two, is on the island but in Palma with his partner in a new business importing Indonesian furniture into Spain. I give them some details of the past year and the challenges of the "cancer twins" and how blessed I feel to be participating in another magical summer with my family and friends.

The next day, I stop by Kevin's housekeeper's house in Pollença for my stuff, about eight boxes. I don't own a home on the island, but over many renting years, I have accumulated things to add personal touches to our summer dwelling and satisfy my nesting instinct: dishes, glasses, bowls, pitchers, coffee pot, and linens. I store them for the rest of the year in Amalia's garage and give her a nice present.

Once my boxes are loaded, I head toward the sea, to the Port of Pollença, around the edge of the Bay of Pollença, to the town of

Alcúdia where I used to live. As I circle the city of Alcúdia, I can see the remains of my father's Roman city, Pollentia, on the outskirts to the right. The present-day city of Pollença, where I have just been, is twenty minutes away, inland. The Roman domination of Mallorca ended in the third century AD. Having lost her military power, the city was invaded by vandals. The Pollentians fled inland to the hills, resettled, and kept the name of their former town. As I pass by, I see the remainder of a row of Roman marble columns reconstructed along a market street in the center of the excavation. I hope my body can be reconstructed to a healthy state as well, and I look forward to the renewed energy a month in paradise will provide. I continue to drive around Alcúdia and out to the small beach community called Mal Pas, meaning "bad way" or "bad road" in Mallorquin, the local language.

My excitement builds as I head down the last bit of road towards our house. Suddenly I see the sea, our sea, the lush, turquoise glow of the Mediterranean intensified by the August sun. I make the last turn down our hill and see the house called *El Barco* in front of me. The house is aptly named "The Boat." The main part of the cream, stucco structure is a round tower with two rows of large round windows up and downstairs facing the sea.

All across the front of the house are patios for dining, sunning, and sitting to read or watch the boats coming and going from the small marina to the right. Daniel, his girlfriend, Anne, and their close friends, Scott and Elizabeth, are already at the house. We divide chores and trips to gather supplies and regroup to assemble our first salad lunch outside with the spectacular views.

After the sacred siesta in my upstairs tower room, I go outside and walk to the edge of the property on the left and look across to the crescent beach filled with sun worshippers on towels and lounge chairs. I remember the years I would come out at noon and watch for my father, who would come to the beach, sit on his towel, and lather up. His thick head of wavy, white hair was red in his youth, and his freckled skin belonged in the Ireland of his ancestors, not the hot Mediterranean. He would get toasty for about fifteen minutes and then

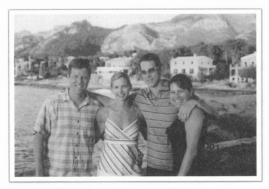

Scott, Elizabeth, Daniel, and Anne in Mallorca.

make his way quickly over the hot sand and slowly into the cool water. I would swim out from the rocks below me and meet him in the middle of the little bay. We would tread water and talk of summer things: his finds of the morning on the dig, the friends I had dined with the night before. We continued the ritual until his last summer near the sea at the age of eighty-five. I wonder how often he thought about the rituals that would be passed on, the rituals so ingrained in my identity. I have been swimming in this water since I was thirteen. The Spanish saltwater mingles with my blood, like a good drug, a healing drug. The sea represents the part of me that is alive and well, the place where child-hood memories never die and new memories are stored, memories for my children. Given the strong chemo drugs necessary to fight my horrible cancer, I wonder how close I will make it to my father's eighty-five years. I vow to enjoy each moment of the rest of the summer.

Our first night together, Daniel, his friends, and I walk up the hill to the small restaurant El Cocodrillo, eat chipirones (baby squid fried in a light batter) with lemon, and share light catch-up conversation with the owners. And then the conversation turns more serious. Doctor Daniel wants details about my health and his father's health, and how we are faring the aftermath of all the zappings. I am pleased to give him only good reports, and we toast to the joy of good news in our favorite place on earth. And we toast memories of our youngest son, Matthew, who usually entertains us after dinner on the terrace. We toast our oldest, Jamie, and his family who are with us this summer only in spirit.

The next day, I drive back to Palma to pick up Jim, and the rest of the week is filled with family gatherings and dinners and laughter and a celebration of wellness. The weather is unusually cool for August. My large collection of scarves will perhaps be tolerable.

I am nervous about the hair issue for the first outing on Kevin's old Mallorcan fishing boat, called a *llaut*. He keeps it at the marina near our house and takes it out for a picnic lunch at least twice a week. My usual drill, diving in and coming up with slicked-back hair, is on hold. After we cross the bay to anchor at a small *calla* (cove) for our first picnic lunch, I climb down the steps instead of diving in and the scarf gets wet in the back, and so what? I can't bring myself to bare my bald head, even with just family. With the twenty extra pounds that didn't drop off as they were supposed to, I would look like a Buddha.

We kiss the kids goodbye on Friday morning and Jim drives back to Palma to pick up Dana and Carole, and our week of party arrangements begins.

Dana, Carole, and I spend the first week gathering cotton bandanas (I don't want anyone to feel left out), brochures, watercolors, brushes, and paper cut into four-by-six inch pieces, all to be stuffed into Mallorcan-straw welcome baskets. Carole sits agile, cross-legged on the floor with her short, curly red hair a clue to her feisty personality, bitching over and over about how she and Dana didn't get a basket, "We're just poor workers." "And I expect you to do a watercolor anyway," I add. Dana, blond and slender, breaks into her perfect smile showing legendary white teeth, "I already have mine started."

The next day, Kevin, Barbara, and their son Alexander come for lunch with Caroline, an old English friend who also grew up in Mallorca, staying with her grandmother each summer. I can still picture her grandmother, sitting with a gin tonic and a cigarette in a holder at the Brisas Bar in the Port of Pollença, her white hair in a bun, her tall, slender body draped in a white cotton dress, accessorized with oversized, aqua flower earrings and strappy, high-heeled sandals in the exact same tone. She would look down at me with stern, piercing eyes and in a deep, cigarette voice, quiz me about school. The importance of being with friends who knew me as a child, whose family knew my parents and my history, is affirming after my year of drugs. The only childhood friends that I have kept up with are on this remote island in Spain.

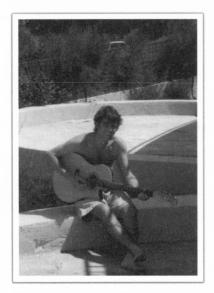

Matthew entertaining us on the terrace in Mallorca.

Caroline has always been an exotic beauty, like her grandmother, living an intriguing life. Her first husband was a mysterious, wealthy Persian who was raised in England. Her second husband was one of the heirs to a large food company in England. Caroline has been part of my e-mail team and again I feel a new dimension slipping into another friendship. Just as I experienced at home, I am particularly conscious about something special happening with old Mallorcan friends. Their empathy and support continuously surprise me in a wondrous way during my path to healing. The onset of a life-threatening illness ratchets up the connection we share.

Over the next week, Jim, Carole, Dana, and I visit the restaurants where we have tentatively reserved three tables of ten for Tuesday through Thursday night.

British friends Christine and Tony have arrived early and rented a house between Alcúdia and Pollença for their whole family for two weeks. Christine is another childhood friend from London whose family used to summer in Mal Pas, and both she and Tony are lawyers. Their youngest daughter, Emily, is my godchild.

On Monday of the birthday week, Claudie and Doug arrive from Paris. Doug is a larger-than-life, bon vivant who practices securities law like Jim and lived in Nashville for a few years. He is godfather to our youngest son, Matthew. He has lived in France for fifteen years with his second wife, Claudie, who is French and also a lawyer. The quieter moments with a few old friends before the whole crowd arrives set a celebratory tone.

This morning I awake at four, the first restless night since my arrival. I am too excited to sleep. Our bed faces the semicircle of four, round windows like the prow of a ship. On either side are two doors, opened to allow a cross-breeze flow. Now the air is still after two days of unusual wind and cool weather, but with my head always

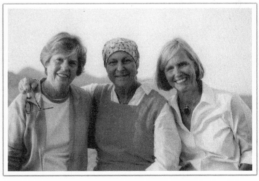

Siggy with her handmaidens, Carole and Dana.

covered, I am just as glad to have a respite from the usual heat. I look out over the jagged rocks beyond the cove to my left to see the outline of Manresa, the oldest house in Mal Pas. Behind the dramatic silhouette of this old house and the surrounding king palm trees, we watch the nightly sunsets. Out the other door, I see the pink glow from the sunrise over La Victoria Mountain behind the marina on the other side of the cove. The full drama from daybreak to sunset can be seen from my recumbent position in bed or anywhere on the patio, the beginning and end of each day from ship's prow. I never tire of the daily dance, the interplay of sun and clouds constantly painting a changing picture at the opening and closing of each day.

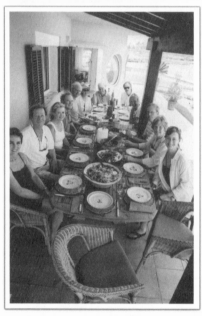

Lunch on the terrace of "El Barco."
Clockwise from left: Jennie, Tony, Pat, Steve,
James, Carol, Siggy, Keith, Dana, John,
Carole, and Linda.

How many spots on earth offer a balanced view of both spectacles?

Today the marathon begins. Two years in the planning, the once-in-a-lifetime celebration that has kept me focused through four months of chemo is about to play out.

The next twenty or so guests arrive by Tuesday, a few in time for lunch on our terrace. Doug, with his new bandana around his neck, and Claudie help host, arriving with a newly purchased blender and the ingredients for fresh cucumber soup, another recipe shared from their extensive, post-retirement travels. My collection of Mallorcan pottery bowls are filled with local salads like trampo, finely diced tomatoes, onions, and mild pale-green peppers. The wooden cheese tray is heaped with Mahon cheeses in various states of aging, mild to sharp. A bottle of rosado wine is open at each end of the table. The local brown bread and the Mallorcan dried biscuits called *galletas* are together in an olive wood bowl. The flavors mix with the gentle breeze off the sea and the tired, yet exhilarated voices of the newly arrived.

By Wednesday, most of the group assemble for the first planned drinks and dinner at La Victoria Restaurant, nestled into the mountain above our house and overlooking the crescent of lights across the Bay of Pollença, where the Port of Pollença is coming to life. Electricity is in the air. As I breathe in the joy of this gathering, I pray my birthday gift will include a return to com-

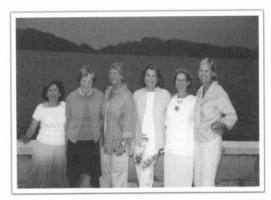

My magnificent friends on the wall. From left: Connie, Carole, Siggy, Anne, Anne Taylor, and Dana.

plete health and many more gatherings and memories with these treasured friends in the years to come.

Thursday morning, I roll over in bed and watch the surface of the water below me in constant motion, ripples moving towards the shore where they gently crash, turning into white bubbles against the jagged black rocks around the cove. The sky is grey when I step outside and take the car into Alcúdia for fresh bread. The rain came down in sheets last night. Rain is rare in August. People here comment when there is a cloud in the sky. What is going on? Maybe the cooler temperature is Mother Nature's birthday gift to the scarf queen.

By noon, the sky is back to a cloudless blue. The unusual light is like spring: crisp and clear as glass. The rain from the night before has washed away the haze that usually rises from the dark, rocky coast's constant exposure to hot, penetrating sun. Another eight guests come for a swim at our beach and lunch. Just as we finish lunch around three-thirty, the last two couples arrive, and we set out more salad. The meal continues until five-thirty, a new record.

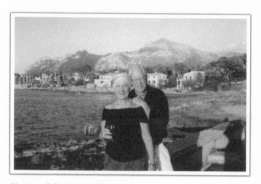

Siggy and Jim in Mallorca.

Dinner in the square in Pollença at the trendy Il Giardino Restaurant, under the oversized, white umbrellas, is over too quickly. I wish I could slow down time. And then Doug does. He arrives the next morning with pictures of each table from last night mounted on a poster board with a picture of me in the center. One of his new gadgets is a portable photo printer. Even with all activities accelerated by the wind, I will be able to treasure my many pictures.

The Friday night alfresco dinner at El Barco, hosted by our houseguests, features a Mallorcan ratatouille, called *tumbet*, from a nearby restaurant.

Just before the guests arrive, Dana reverently hands me the water-color she has been slaving over all week. She has created an exact floor plan of the downstairs of our house with all the furniture, and including the rental car with the back window smashed from backing into an olive tree (I didn't do it) and the broken rocking chair stashed in the corner of the garage. Carole flips her fifteen-minute, marker cartoon across the table. Her French-blue bathing suit with a tightly cinched-in waist fills one side of the paper and an Indian silk blouse, locally acquired, fills the other side. A caption reads, *Dos outfitos.*

As people come in, they hand me their watercolors and I display them around the crescent of windows in the living room. They are imaginative, diverse, with a liberal use of bright blues, yellows, pinks. I am spellbound by the collective talent of the group, especially the men. I had thought I would receive one painting from each couple at best, but in many cases, both produced incredible works: views of the sea and boats, windmills, a patio, a typical Mallorcan doorway. The endless, picturesque vistas in Alcúdia and the nearby countryside bring out the dormant muses. My favorite is Steve's view of a clock tower from their hotel bedroom. In the lower, right-hand corner he has signed it and then added in pencil: 10 euros. I am already imagining a wall in our Florida house hung with my gifts.

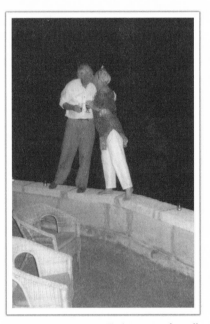

Jim's toast on the wall.

After dinner, all of my women friends stand in front of the wall by the water, draped in pink and aqua and yellow boas matching their bright blouses and swaying skirts—no blacks and beiges in this group—and serenade me with a song to the tune of "Hello Dolly" written in anticipation of the trip with input from Nicky and her daughter, my other goddaughter, Craig. Kevin reads a poem he has composed. Carole H. has even written a song in Spanish that Anne's husband, Bill, sings.

Then Jim jumps up on the wall and pulls me up to join him. He looks handsome, his slender body dressed in a white linen shirt and beige linen pants, his grey hair in a new, closely cropped style. He thanks our friends for coming, toasts Kevin and Barbara, thanks

Carole and Dana for all their hard work. He talks about the legacy of my father and the important role he played in our being in this place. Then he speaks about the last five months and the challenges we have both endured that give such depth to the celebration. Jim talks about seeing traits in me he never knew I had. He talks about being in awe

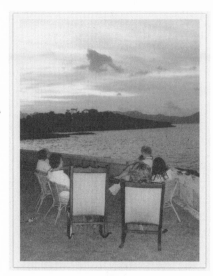

Gathering at sunset at "El Barco."

of the way I handled the news of cancer and the endless decisions that followed. He talks about how much he loves me, how he thinks I am a remarkable woman. In front of all the people I love most, Jim speaks of things we rarely cover in private. People weep, I weep.

On Saturday morning, we tour the small museum in Alcúdia, where the treasures from the excavation are displayed: selections of pottery, amphora, coins, fishing hooks, glass, and jewelry. My favorite piece of art is an exquisite bronze head, about ten inches high, of a young Roman girl with a patrician profile and artfully arranged curls. I remember the excitement of the find when I was a young girl of about the same age. The sculpture was discovered at the bottom of a well where it must have been tossed to avoid detection by invaders, perhaps right before the inhabitants were forced to flee to the hills of present day Pollença. The plan worked for close to two thousand years.

The peak of the celebration is Saturday night when we take over Es Convent Restaurant in Alcúdia for the final dinner. Tonight we include a selection of friends who have summer homes in Mallorca.

I sit next to Luis, a friend from Madrid, for the first and second course and then switch with Dana and sit at another table next to another Mallorcan friend for dessert.

Luis and his wife, Tissa, are two of my favorite summer people. Tissa has a significant collection of succulents in her garden and has inspired my own start of a similar quest. Clippings from some of Tissa's succulents are thriving as two-and three-year-old plants in my Nashville garden. I guess I'm guilty of another herbaceous crime, smuggling live material out of Spain.

On Sunday morning, most of our guests leave. Jim and I sit with our feet up on the seawall where he had made his toast. Yesterday's rain has again cleared the air, and the outline of black jagged mountains across the bay appear as sharp as a razor's edge and blacker than pitch.

We are reluctant to vacate our special spot, but Barbara and Kevin are hosting a lunch for the few guests who are staying through Sunday night. For the final group meal, we sit around an oval table under the rose arbor on their terrace, set with green-tinted wine glasses and green pottery bowls filled with pink gazpacho. Surrounding us are olive, carob, fig, and lemon trees and the mountains beyond. We sit and eat and rehash the week, and I try to hold the magic in my heart just a little longer.

Jim leaves on Monday morning and I move in with Barbara and Kevin for the last week of the month, another ritual I see now as a sacred part of my yearly routine—a concentrated visit with my brother and sister-in-law. I give my house to Alexander, allowing the younger generation to enjoy our house on the sea. The soothing rhythms and simple routines of Barbara and Kevin's summer house, the last quiet week without guests, is better than a spa and holds fonder memories with each passing year.

My last full day, the weather turns warm again, and Barbara, Kevin, and I go out for a last spin in the old llaut. We slow down in front of El Barco and watch Alexander and his business partner, Rafa, assemble one of their teak gazebo beds from Indonesia on the lawn of our house. They are having an open house tonight and have invited all the locals to view their wares. Our boat moves around in a circle and heads out past the large villas set in the cliffs beyond the marina, past the children's camp called La Victoria, past the restaurant by the same name where we had our first joint dinner, and out to our favorite cove, Las Caletas, for the final picnic lunch of the summer. The mountain La Victoria rises above us, made from the same black rock as in front of our house. Barbara and I hiked to the top a few years ago and the spectacular view stays in my memory bank. From the top, you can see any approaching ship for many miles and into the Bay of Pollença on the left or the Bay of Alcúdia on the right. The natural lookout was one of the reasons this site was chosen for the city of Pollentia several thousand years ago. We arrive at the cove and count about thirty boats already anchored, the largest ones farther out. Our five-and-a-half-meter boat maneuvers into a space near the beach.

As soon as we settle in and drop anchor, a voice greets us from the water, an Italian acquaintance of Kevin's, Sergio. He hangs on the ladder that we have just put in place and chats for a few minutes. Kevin invites him onboard for a beer. "No, no, I better not. I'm naked. I hate to swim in trunks." And as he swims swiftly away a few minutes later, we see that he isn't naked; he is wearing fins, bright yellow. Any more interesting bits are lost under the ripples of the sea.

We follow our usual boat drill. First we set up the *toldo*, a flat, canvas cover that rolls out five feet above the top of the boat. As we roll out the canvas, Kevin supervises from the stern, calling for a tighter tie on the left, then a tighter tie on the right, four ties on each side until the six-foot cover shades most of the boat and is balanced in a perfect parallel with the sea. The lines on the bow and stern of the boat that are used to tie up at the marina are rolled into perfect, flat snakelike coils, called Flemish flakes. Revarnished and painted each winter, my brother's boat—and my brother, for that matter—are always shipshape.

When the canopy is secured, we all go in for a swim. My scarf causes me to again use the ladder. Barbara and I tread water and she speaks enthusiastically about our friends, whom she has now spent enough time with to know better than before, and the meals that we shared.

Back on board, we open wine and start to set up lunch. Two older matrons have just dropped into the water from the small boat to our left. I pick up their distinctive Madrid accent but soon lose the conversation as the two ladies drift farther out and talk too fast. Barbara starts to laugh to herself. "*¿Que pasa?*" I ask. Barbara explains that the woman to the right, in a white bathing suit with red roses, is a renowned fashion diva who often will fly to Paris for the day to buy clothes. Her son is studying for the priesthood. Everyone in Madrid knows how upset she is about this fate for her only son, but he is about to take his final vows and she is making the best of the situation. She is concerned about how he will be dressed for the ceremony and where he will have his set of vestments made. She wonders if their regular tailor in Madrid could make them. The other woman, in blue, thinks that they probably need to be made by a tailor who specializes in the intricate details of church vestments. After a few more stokes and a few more exchanged possibilities, the blue bathing suit says, "Hell, why don't you just call the Pope and find out who his tailor is in Rome?" Ah, the absurdity of details people obsess over when nothing serious fills their horizon.

Barbara and I set out the vine-ripe tomatoes, fresh brown bread, olive oil, and salt for *pan con tomate*, the perfect summer lunch at sea when the tomatoes and bread and summer breezes are just right. I slice bread and give thanks for this small part of the Mediterranean that is so much a part of me.

That evening at sunset, we make an appearance at the open house hosted by Alexander and Rafa at our Mal Pas house. The gazebo bed is striking set up in the corner of the garden lawn, looking out on the next point where the oldest house, Manresa, stands before the setting sun. I lie down in the square, teak sofa bed with pillow rolls at both ends and four, wood posts that support a black umbrella-like roof. The sunset from this angle is fresh and new. Other teak furniture—chairs and benches and tables—are dotted around the lawn. People mill around in summer party clothes, and I catch up with some of the old Mal Pas crowd whom I haven't seen all summer.

Homeward Bound

*T*he next morning I awake at 6:00 AM, then 6:30, then 6:45, the way one does when about to travel. I am dressed and my hand luggage is packed when the alarm goes off at 7:00. The big bags are already in my rental car. I take a bottle of water, a small bag of *guiettas*, and ease out of the narrow drive and down the equally narrow road banked on both sides by dry-stacked stone walls and other restored farmhouses. The rising sun is low on the horizon in front of me, but will soon be behind me when I turn onto the main road to cross the island to Palma. Even at 7:00 AM the traffic is bumper-to-bumper between Pollença and the middle of the island where the motorway begins. Construction trucks are working every dozen yards or so along the side of the road, creating a major devastation, destroying old walls, old trees, and exposing huge tracts of red soil. By next summer, the motorway will reach Pollença and Alcúdia. I will miss the narrow road, dry-stacked stone walls, plane trees, and stone farmhouses in close proximity, the road close enough to watch the workers in the fields harvesting crops, like something out of a French Impressionist painting. Part of the ritual of arrival and departure each summer is touching the farm life for a moment on the way to the sea, counting off the few remaining towns we now pass through that will be lost. I will not miss the bumper-to-bumper traffic and the huge buses as slow as snails.

As I poke along behind one now, I reflect back on dozens of past Mallorca vacations, confirming that a month is the perfect amount of time. I am ready to return home and begin the next chapter, whatever it may be.

In the car, I think about the scheduled next round of chemo in two days. I can't believe that after increased energy, after feeling almost normal, after seeing the beginnings of black fur on my scalp, I may need to plunge back into sick mode. Fresh from the aqua-blue sea, my tan body cannot leave the mindset of my Spanish life, even though I clearly remember Dr. Greer's "Let's just schedule the procedure in case" scenario happening just before I left for Spain. I know chemo number five is in the Vanderbilt system, scheduled for the morning of August 30.

I cannot turn my mind from the ripe memories of a Spanish summer, a magical summer, a healthy summer. On the trip home—on the planes from Palma to Madrid, Madrid to New York, New York to Nashville—I keep my mind on the long, lazy lunches; the daily siestas with the slap of the sea; the afternoon reads on the patio; the market days with straw baskets filled with fruits and lettuces and tomatoes; breathing in the smell of fresh-baked bread while standing in line at the bakery; sampling the perfect Mahon cheese at the butcher before he wraps it in white wax paper and asks, "¿Algo mas?" (Anything else?); the looks on my friends' faces the first time they step through the door of our patio and view the sea beyond; drinking cocktails with our feet up on the wall looking out at the boats on the bay; looking over the outline of the Manresa mansion against the setting sun; the morning rooster; and the church bell before Saturday afternoon and Sunday morning mass. Maybe if I had these experiences for more than just one month each year, they would lose their magic. Maybe the anticipation of arrival and the inevitable departure each August keep both the memories from my youth and the layers I keep adding in a perpetual state of freshness, even with contemplation of next summer's completion of the motorway.

Do I really have to go back to being "Patient Siggy"? When Dr. Greer said, "That doesn't mean it won't come back," did he mean now? Will there be any lump when he probes under my arms on Tuesday? Will I lose my black peach fuzz? Again?

My wig is rolled up in a small ball in one of my scarves. I never wore it in Mallorca. Not once. I put it on a few times in front of the mirror, but always took it off again. I passed it around after lunch one day, and Daniel and his friends tried it on—I have the pictures to prove it. But the wig never seemed to fit into island life.

As I lift off on the runway at LaGuardia for the last leg home, I close my eyes and recite my ritual Our Father lift-off prayer. I try to move back into the mode of calm I experienced before chemo one, when the circle of friends at home and their unified prayers seemed to be assuring me that God was close, but I can't find that place.

I have one day to recover from the trip before the next hospital visit. The whirlwind summer and long ride home catch up, and once in the house, my bags remain open on the dressing-room floor, unpacked.

Facing the Music

$\mathcal{O}$n Tuesday, August 30, I go to Dr. Greer's office instead of straight to the first floor of the Vanderbilt Clinic for chemo. I need blood work and a chance to touch base with Dr. Greer before knowing how to proceed. When I arrive at the hematology department on the second floor of the Vanderbilt Clinic, I sit in the waiting room and fill out the usual forms. Rank my pain on a scale of 1 to 10: 0, 0, 0. What has changed since my last visit? I have turned into a well person again. When I was in the routine of chemo last spring and early summer, I was handling it. But coming back to talk about two more chemos is like starting sick mode from scratch, as if I had never been there in the first place. How could I so easily forget? Then I remembered from years past how quickly the pain of childbirth was forgotten.

Marsha takes my blood pressure. It is high again. Is that because I am nervous or because I have not had poisons in me for more than six weeks? In addition to other things, the chemo keeps my blood pressure down. Marsha sticks a short, fat needle into my port and draws the eight vials of blood. An examination room is ready, and I go in and sit. Dr. Greer knocks right away, five minutes early. Jim is not here yet and I need him to be here. Dr. Greer examines all the places where lymph nodes can enlarge: my arms, my neck, my collar-bone, my groin. No lumps.

I can't help revisiting the main issues, re-asking the same questions, "Why do I need more treatment? The tests show I am clear and

I feel great. If there is a strong chance that another cancer could come back and since I need to have all the good cells possible to continue to fight my chronic CLL condition, why wouldn't it be better to take a pass on more chemo?" In my mind I am also thinking about my newly sprouted black fuzz, but keep it to myself.

Dr. Greer repeats that the standard profile for cancer is two more treatments even after no sign of cancer is visible. He confirms that the standard profile of a patient with CLL is a recurrence of some form of cancer within eighteen months to three years. Even with my good reports, experience shows there could be cancer-lurking cells below the radar screen undetected by the PET scan. He goes on, "I would have to recommend the additional two treatments." Then he tilts his head up, looks me in the eye for just a second and gives me his shy smile, "But I could be talked out of it." I say, "Would I regret not doing two more if the cancer comes back?" He just looks at me and says nothing. We both know it is my call. Finally, I say, "I'm going to go with whatever you recommend. I'm in your hands."

Then Jim arrives. Dr. Greer does a short recap. I think I have made a decision, but when Jim turns into the devil's advocate, I am glad. I see his point, too. Before embarking on more treatment, I need to be sure. Jim counters with saving the chemo guns for the possibility of a next round. CHOP+R is so powerful that it can be administered to the patient only so many times. To the question of how many, which has been asked before, Dr. Greer reminds us—about ten. Seeing Jim's argument, I continue to push, "Wouldn't I be wasting my big guns while I am in a healthy state?"

I thought I had made up my mind and then Jim changed it. Even though the plan is on hold again, I welcome Jim's view. We come at illness in different ways but respect each other's differences. My mother used to say, "A crisis will make you or break you." The struggles of the last year have deepened Jim's and my relationship, and I am grateful for another gift.

Dr. Greer suggests additional blood analysis to track blood flow. If the CLL is also in remission, we would not do more chemo. If some trace remains, we would do another bone-marrow biopsy next week.

Marsha sticks my port again for another six vials. The second time really hurts. Dr. Greer will call tomorrow. More waiting. More decisions. I leave more stressed than I have been since the first month of diagnosis. I am back in a holding pattern, waiting to see if the CLL cancer cells floating somewhere in my system will flare up and be noticed. The Richter's is gone, isn't it? My stomach is churning and I feel the anxiety I thought I had shed last May.

We are supposed to keep Jack and Baker for a few hours while Jamie and Lisa go for dinner, but I just can't do it. My energy is zapped. I need time to vegetate, draw on inner resources, be alone, pour a strong drink, recover from the jet lag. Not seeing enough of my grandchildren is a major downside of my treatments, but what could I do? I would just have to make it up later. The indecision about how to proceed is the worst. I take my Mallorca clothes out of the big duffel bag, pile them again on the dressing-room floor and stash the luggage upstairs. One step accomplished.

Dr. Greer calls and the "sheets" of affected cells in my blood are no longer there, but I still have traces of bad cells. He recommends the bone-marrow biopsy.

The following week, I go in for the second bone-marrow biopsy, the twilight sleep, the bed recovery, the few days wait for the results. Thank God that Ellen, Dr. Greer's nurse-practitioner, does most of the bone-marrow biopsies at Vanderbilt and is renowned for her special touch.

Again Dr. Greer calls to say the cancer cells are way down from last spring, but some remain, and he recommends the additional two chemos. By now, I am ready. A compromise is the elimination of the most deadly drug, Adriamycin or the "red devil," and we schedule the first of the last two chemos for September 9, two weeks from the originally scheduled date. "Did I lose ground by waiting for so long for these last two?" I ask. "I don't think so," Dr. Greer assures me.

Chemo Five

On September 8, Ellen goes over my medications and comes in puzzled about a discrepancy in the dosage for the prednisone, a steroid I take for five days after the chemo, but I am still preoccupied with my decision to have the two more chemos and not paying too much attention. She says for some reason she can't get a 100 mg tablet, so it is important to remember to take two of the 50 mg tablets she has ordered. I agree and go home, picking up all my prescriptions on the way. At home I look at the old bottle of prednisone I had taken during the first four chemos and the prescription was for a 20 mg tablet. How could the dosage have been so off? I decide that the 20 mg tablet worked just fine for the first four chemos, so I take only one 50 mg pill for the following five days. Then I get in bed with my laptop and start working on the next "Patient Siggy" update. I need my troops, now numbering 160, on board.

UPDATE FROM PATIENT SIGGY
SEPTEMBER 10, 2005
DEAR FRIENDS,

AUGUST IN MALLORCA TOPS MY LIST OF MAJOR MEMORIES. SUMMERS ON THIS MAGICAL ISLAND ARE A RITUAL IN MY LIFE AS STRONG AS CHRISTMAS MORNING AROUND THE TREE, WAITING FOR ALL THE FAMILY TO ARRIVE BEFORE OPENING PRESENTS. I LIKE TO SAY THAT HALF OF MY SOUL LIVES IN SPAIN. PLANNING THE NEXT AUGUST IN MALLORCA IS WHAT I THINK ABOUT FOR THE REST OF THE YEAR. MALLORCA DEFINES A PART OF ME, WHERE MY CHILD-HOOD MEMORIES LIVE, WHERE I WALK THE STREETS I WALKED WITH

MY FATHER, WHERE I CAN SHARE LEISURELY LUNCHES WITH MY BROTHER AND SISTER-IN-LAW, KEVIN AND BARBARA, THEIR BOYS, OUR BOYS. NO ONE IS IN A HURRY AND CONVERSATIONS ARE RARELY CUT SHORT.

MANY NASHVILLE FRIENDS HAVE JOINED US FOR VISITS OVER THE YEARS BUT NEVER AS MANY AS THIS YEAR, WHEN I INVITED A LARGER GROUP FOR A MUCH-PLANNED SIXTIETH BIRTHDAY CELEBRATION. I DIDN'T KNOW TWO YEARS AGO, WHEN THE EVENT WAS FIRST CONCEIVED, THAT WE WOULD BE CELEBRATING THE JOYOUS NEWS OF THE DISAPPEARANCE OF THE BIG-CELL LYMPHOMA I HAD BEEN FIGHTING WITH MASSIVE DOSES OF CHEMO SINCE APRIL.

FROM AUGUST 1, WHEN I ARRIVED AT OUR IDYLLIC HOUSE BY THE SEA, I WAS ON A HIGH. THE FIRST WEEK, OUR MIDDLE SON, DANIEL, HIS GIRLFRIEND, ANNE, AND ANOTHER YOUNG COUPLE, SCOTT AND ELIZABETH, SHARED THE HOURS WITH JIM AND ME. AS TRADITION DICTATED, EACH DAY CENTERED AROUND LUNCHES ON THE TERRACE OVERLOOKING THE MEDITERRANEAN, WATCHING THE BOAT PARADE, EATING SPANISH CHEESES, MAHON, MANCHEGO, WITH BIG SALADS, FRESH VEGGIES, BROWN BREAD BAKED THAT MORNING, AND ROSADO WINE (A LIGHT ROSE ONLY DRINKABLE IN SPAIN, IN SUMMER), FOLLOWED BY A TWO-HOUR SIESTA.

THE SECOND WEEK CAROLE AND DANA ARRIVED TO HELP PLAN THE CELEBRATION FOR WEEK THREE. THEY DUBBED THEMSELVES "THE HAND MAIDENS" AND WENT TO WORK ORGANIZING WELCOME BASKETS AND DINNERS TO BE SHARED EACH NIGHT.

THAT WEEK OF QUIET CAMARADERIE AND PREPARATION— WALKING TO SIMPLE RESTAURANTS NEARBY FOR DINNER, SHARING MOMENTS FROM PAST SUMMERS WITH A FEW GUESTS WHO CAME EARLY—WAS MAYBE THE BEST PART OF THE SUMMER. THE ANTICIPA-TION OF THE GREAT WEEK TO COME, FAT WITH PROMISE, WAS SHARED BY ALL.

THE WEEK OF THE BIRTHDAY CELEBRATION WENT BY IN A FLASH. I COULDN'T HOLD ON TO THE MULTIPLE MOMENTS I WANTED TO FREEZE. THANK GOODNESS FOR A DOZEN VERSIONS OF DIGITAL CAMERAS AND ESPECIALLY, THE ONE HOLDOUT THAT HAS TO WAIT FOR A VISIT TO WOLF CAMERA UPON REENTRY, JIM'S CRISP SHOTS FROM HIS MINOLTA MAXXUM 7. WHAT BETTER HAPPINESS COULD FILL MY HEART THAN TO SHARE MY SACRED PLACE WITH SPECIAL FRIENDS? I ONLY WISH MORE FRIENDS COULD HAVE BEEN INCLUDED.

The last week I spent with Kevin and Barbara, resting, recovering, reminiscing. Our last week together, just family, has become another treasured part of my summer ritual.

All August I was a well person, a happy celebrant without a care except for the weather, which was never too hot. My focus for the past spring was curing the big cancer, the hateful Richter's syndrome with the big, scary diagnosis. And we did it, and I do mean we: doctors, prayers, embracing friends. The sucker was gone. *Gracias a Dios.*

I had given little thought to reentry to Nashville and the next step, the two more chemos left, scheduled way beyond the horizon I could see each day from the patio dining table. The little thought I let sneak in was OK, I'm cured, surely more chemo was overkill. I had to live with the other chronic leukemia still hovering in my bloodstream and bone marrow. More chemo would further damage my body that needed to fight the CLL that was destined to be a companion for the rest of my life.

So I came home, happy but exhausted, jet-lagged, feeling every inch of my sixty years taking a greater toll on changing time zones and long plane rides, even from the front of the bus. Jim has lots of air miles.

I unpacked my oversized bag and promptly put it away in the deep closet upstairs. Then my efficiency collapsed. My stacks of clothes, my stash of books and papers, my pastel espadrilles, and my eight jars of green mustard (that you really should be able to get here and let me know if you find it) stayed in piles on the floor of my dressing room for two weeks. My unread e-mails hit three figures. I took naps. I watched CNN. I read my novel. I somehow couldn't return phone messages, write in my journal, or organize my selection of digital Kodak summer pictures. I was frozen. I was a big lump. My bed was my best friend.

Jim and I met with Dr. Greer. He recommended the standard procedure after a cancer "cure": two more treatments. Then he looked up with his shy, engaging smile and said, "But I could be talked out of it." I knew that Jim was leaning toward no more chemo. The two

STRONG OPINIONS I COUNTED ON MOST WERE ON OPPOSITE SIDES OF THE SMALL EXAMINATION ROOM. WE DECIDED TO RUN MORE TESTS, TAKE MORE BLOOD, PROBABLY DO ANOTHER BONE-MARROW BIOPSY, AND THINK. THERE WAS NO RIGHT OR WRONG ANSWER IN MY CASE. MY LITTLE BODY (BIGGER AFTER ALL THAT CHEESE AT LUNCH), WOULD BE SUBJECTED TO MORE TESTS. WE WOULD HAVE A WEEK TO WAIT FOR THE RESULTS, CONSIDER THE ALTERNATIVES; I COULD STRESS AND THEN WE WOULD MEET AGAIN.

AS I DROVE HOME FROM THE VANDERBILT CLINIC, THE FIRST REPORTS FROM THE DEVASTATION FROM HURRICANE KATRINA WERE COMING ACROSS THE AIRWAVES. WAS MY QUANDARY REALLY SO BAD?

MY HAIR WAS GROWING OUT. IT WAS A QUARTER OF AN INCH LONG AT BEST BUT I COULD SEE THE COWLICK IN THE FRONT, BENDING TO THE RIGHT, A PATTERN BEGINNING TO FORM. I COULD RUB MY HAND OVER THE TOP AND FEEL FUZZ INSTEAD OF SKIN. WOULD I GO INTO THE FALL AS A WELL PERSON WITH A NORMAL ROUTINE, ANTICIPATING A HAIR TRIM IN THE FORESEEABLE FUTURE? OR WOULD I MOVE BACK INTO SICK MODE WITH CHEMO ZAPS AND RECOVERIES AND A COLLECTION OF TINY HAIRS EACH MORNING ON MY PILLOW? WHY WAS HAIR SUCH A BIG, DAMN DEAL? WHY DID I HATE MY WIG SO MUCH? I PAID A LOT FOR THAT WIG. I'VE HAD IT CUT THREE TIMES. I TOOK IT TO SPAIN AND NEVER WORE IT. I HAVE A SUPERB COLLECTION OF SCARVES.

I THOUGHT OF MY SIX WEEKS OF CELEBRATION AND WELLNESS AND HAIR GROWTH. HOW COULD I GO BACK? WHEN I WAS IN THE CHEMO ROUTINE OF SPRING AND EARLY SUMMER, I WAS OK. I FOLLOWED A PLAN. I WAS IN A ZONE. I WAS MENTALLY AND SPIRI-TUALLY PRIMED. I WAS SURROUNDED BY MY FRIENDS HOVERING, PEOPLE—HUNDREDS—KEN, MY SPIRITUAL MENTOR, CLAIMED THOUSANDS—WERE PRAYING FOR ME. AFTER THE BIG PRONOUNCE-MENT OF THE CURE, I HAD TOLD THE CHURCH THEY COULD TAKE ME OFF THE PRAYER LIST. HADN'T I DEMANDED ENOUGH OF EVERY-BODY'S TIME? WASN'T IT TIME FOR THEM TO PRAY FOR SOMEONE ELSE? THIS PAST SUNDAY AT CHURCH, I FELT FUNNY, DEFLATED, LEFT OUT. I NEEDED THAT PRAYER LIST MORE THAN EVER AS I MADE THIS DICEY DECISION. AND CRAZY AS IT SOUNDS, BEING OFF THE LIST, I FELT THE DIFFERENCE.

ON THE SECOND VISIT TO DR. GREER, HE CONFIRMED GOOD NEWS FROM THE ADDITIONAL TESTING. THE BIG B-CELL LYMPHOMA

WAS GONE FROM MY BLOOD AND BONE MARROW AND THE CLL WAS DOWN TO TWENTY PERCENT, WAY DOWN FROM THE ORIGINAL DIAGNOSIS. BUT HE WENT ON TO EXPLAIN THAT IN ANY CANCER, THERE COULD BE MORE CELLS IN THE SYSTEM BELOW THE RADAR SCREEN THAT COULD NOT BE DETECTED WITH ANY EXISTING TESTS. THIS WAS WHY A LARGER CANCER COULD RETURN. THIS WAS WHY OVER TIME AND EXPERIENCE, THE PRACTICE OF TWO MORE TREATMENTS AFTER A PRONOUNCED CURE WERE THE STANDARD PROFILE. DR. GREER SAID, "WHY DON'T WE TAKE THE WEEKEND TO THINK ABOUT HOW TO PROCEED? I WILL CONTACT A FEW MORE COLLEAGUES, GET A FEW MORE OPINIONS."

WE AGREED THAT HE WOULD CALL ME ON WEDNESDAY. TODAY. HE SCHEDULED ANOTHER CHEMO FOR THURSDAY, TOMORROW, "JUST IN CASE" WE DECIDED TO GO FOR IT.

LAST SUNDAY AND MONDAY NIGHT I DIDN'T SLEEP. I HAD CONSULTED MY SPECIAL MEDICAL TEAM, DR. JOHN, DR. BILL, AND DR. ROY, FOR ADDITIONAL AMMUNITION. SUNDAY NIGHT, EVEN JIM SAID, "I THINK YOU SHOULD DO THE CHEMO. YOU HAVE TOO MUCH ANXIETY ABOUT THIS AND AREN'T GOING TO BE COMFORTABLE IF YOU TAKE A PASS." AT THAT POINT, I STILL WASN'T SURE. I WAS STILL HOVERING.

BUT BY MONDAY NIGHT I HAD DECIDED. WHO KNOWS WHEN ENOUGH INFORMATION HAS BEEN STORED AND YOU ARE READY TO DECIDE, BUT I KNEW I WAS THERE, THAT I WOULD GO WITH WHAT DR. GREER RECOMMENDED. I KNEW IT WOULD INCLUDE HAIR LOSS. I SCHEDULED LUNCH WITH KEN ON WEDNESDAY. MORE AMMUNITION. THIS AFTERNOON DR. GREER'S OFFICE CONFIRMED IT WAS A GO.

THE GOOD SIDE: SEPTEMBER AND OCTOBER WOULD BE ZAPS AND RECOVERIES BUT ALSO AN EXCUSE FOR KEEPING MY SCHEDULE EMPTY FOR HEALING AND MOST IMPORTANT, WRITING. I DO HOPE THERE IS A BOOK IN HERE SOMEWHERE. DID I TELL YOU? I HAVE A LITERARY AGENT.

I DO STILL NEED YOUR PRAYERS. LOTS. I AM BLESSED BECAUSE OF MY FRIENDS. I COUNT ON ALL OF YOU TO CONTINUE TO SUPPORT ME, JUST A BIT LONGER. AND I AM OH SO GRATEFUL.

HUGS, SIGOURNEY

Within fifteen minutes I have twenty responses and I read them with relish. Each e-mail brings me closer to my audience.

I am stunned by the beauty of my English friend Caroline's reply. She is back on Mallorca:

THIS MORNING I GOT UP KNOWING EXACTLY WHAT I WAS GOING TO DO TO AID YOUR CAUSE. HERE I AM SITTING ON THE ROCKS IN FRONT OF EL BARCO. IT IS QUIET ALL AROUND, IT IS THE LAST DAY OF SUMMER—AND A GLORIOUS DAY IT IS, TOO. THE SEA IS TOTALLY CLEAR AND JUST A LITTLE MOVEMENT ON IT, SO PEACEFUL IT MUST BE HEALING. IF I SIT QUIETLY I CAN HEAR THE ECHOES OF YOUR PARTIES OF THE SUMMER AROUND ME, AND IT JUST FEELS SO HAPPY AND BEAUTIFUL. EARLIER I WENT TO KEVIN'S AND SAT ON THE TERRACE AND I SAID PRAYERS FOR YOU IN BOTH PLACES.

Carole H writes:

YOU ARE AMAZING—WHICH IS NOT A VERY ORIGINAL STATEMENT BECAUSE HUNDREDS OF PEOPLE HAVE ALREADY PROFESSED IT.

MALLORCA WAS THE BEST EVER FOR US. YOU MADE IT COME ALIVE FOR ALL AS BELIEVE ME—NO ONE ELSE COULD HAVE DONE.

THE ABSOLUTE WAS JIM'S TOAST. I WILL NEVER FORGET THE TWO OF YOU ON THE WALL, THE SEA BEHIND YOU—YOU WITH THE TWINKLING TIARA AND JIM FINDING THE WORDS TO EXPRESS THE FEELING THAT WE HAVE ALL HAD EVER SINCE AND EVEN BEFORE THE "THING CALLED CANCER" BEGAN. THE TOAST TO YOU, YOUR LOVE, YOUR BRAVERY, THE TOAST TO YOUR FATHER WERE ALL POWERFUL AND POETIC.

THE SECOND MOST MEMORABLE WAS SIMULTANEOUS AND THAT WAS LOOKING AT KEVIN'S HANDSOME FACE: BEAMING, PROUD, ADORING HIS SISTER SURROUNDED BY HER LOVING FRIENDS.

TRULY I WILL NEVER FORGET THE MAGIC OF THOSE MOMENTS.

And from Jan, whose own triumphs make her responses especially poignant:

I HAVE BEEN THINKING AND WONDERING ABOUT YOU SO MUCH, IMAGINING YOU MAY STILL BE IN SPAIN, CURIOUS ABOUT HOW YOUR

HEALTH IS HOLDING OUT, HOPING I HADN'T BEEN DROPPED FROM
YOUR E-MAIL LIST. IT WAS A NICE LITTLE TRIP I GOT TO TAKE TO
YOUR VACATION PARADISE VIA YOUR WRITING. I COULD FEEL THE
HAIR FUZZ AS I READ ON AND IMAGINED RUBBING MY OWN HEAD AS
IF IT LOOKED LIKE YOU DESCRIBED YOURS AT THIS POINT.

I AM GRATEFUL THE BIG CANCER IS STILL GONE AND NOT
SURPRISED. I KNOW THE PRAYERS, THE DOCS, THE FRIENDS, ETC. ALL
MAKE THAT POSSIBLE BUT YOUR BELIEF—YOUR UNDERSTANDING—
YOUR KNOWING THAT YOU WILL BE OK IS HUGE. I DON'T
UNDERSTAND IT BUT I KNOW THAT MY RECOVERY WAS INEXTRI-
CABLY TIED TO UNDERSTANDING—MY KNOWING THAT I WOULD
WALK AGAIN. AND YOU ARE BLESSED TO HAVE THE CAPACITY TO
FIND THAT, TO HAVE THE ABUNDANT INTERNAL RESOURCES FROM
WHICH TO PULL. THAT'S A GIFT FROM SOMEWHERE.

On September 9, the chemo, minus the "red devil" drug, is more
tolerable than the last four. The recovery is decidedly less severe and
debilitating, and I am definitely less tired without the Adriamycin.
How could the elimination of one drug that is "pushed in" in two
minutes rather than dripped make such a difference? Once I am back
in the chemo zone, am back on the prayer list, and resume my
weekly meetings with Ken, my stress subsides. I wait to see tiny hairs
on my pillow.

Chemo Six

*N*o hairs anywhere but on my head by the time I go back to see Dr. Greer before the final chemo in October. I tell him about checking out the prednisone pills I had taken for the first four chemos and seeing they were 20 mg. Because this dosage seemed to do the trick, I tell him, "I decided to take only one 50 mg pill this round instead of the two that were prescribed." He zaps me with a startled stare. "You were supposed to be taking 100 mg after each treatment from the beginning, and I want you to take 100 mg after this next treatment." "OK, OK." It never occurred to me to check the dosage of a given prescription even though Linda advised me at the very beginning to do so. What would I check it against? The written prescription is handed to the druggist and not returned, or the prescription is called in and has no paper trail. I just pick up the pills and follow the instructions: take one a day for five days. I should have paid more attention to Linda's early advice and gotten a written sheet on all drugs and their dosages. Next time. I look through the notebook Linda gave me right after my diagnosis, and the only written paper regarding prednisone was a prescription sheet for 20 mgs. I wonder why I still had the prescription sheet and how it had been filled without being turned in, but I couldn't remember any other details. Would the lower voltage of prednisone affect my cure? Somehow, I didn't think so. My strong body handled the powerful zaps and I would handle the lesser dosage.

Update from Patient Siggy

October 7, 2005

Dearest Friends,

Here we go again. Last time, and I am still preoccupied with hair. Dr. Greer says I will lose it again but so far nothing on my pillow, on the shower floor.

My hair has been growing since Mallorca, with the suspension of chemo since the middle of July. I like to think sea air, pure Spanish olive oil, Manchego cheese, fresh vegetables from the Sunday market, and Mediterranean sun are totally responsible for stimulating hair follicles.

I noticed this morning that the hair on the top of my head, which is twice as thick as the hair on the sides, has assumed a forward position, almost a precursor to bangs I could flip. Wait, that's an exaggeration, but I can slightly alter the little suckers, up, down. I stare at men with short cuts in the checkout line of Harris Teeter and imagine the possibilities in a few more months.

I'm waiting for my new stubble to fall out and trying to remember exactly when my hair started falling out before. How can a quarter inch of hair, a black scalp instead of white, be such a deal? Is it a symbol of healing? A friend who is also undergoing chemo for leukemia and has not lost her hair told me to try a dietary supplement called "cell food" that adds oxygen to every cell in your body. I remember the importance of deep breathing and figure I'll give it a shot. I go to Wild Oats and talk to the tall man with the white beard who hangs out in the vitamin department, and he highly recommends it as well.

I have been the scarf queen all summer, my expensive wig sitting on its Styrofoam head, neglected. Having my head constantly covered is claustrophobic. I am halfway through *Reading* Lolita *in Tehran.* Why don't all those fanatic Arab men walk around in chadors or bhurkas for a week or so and see how they like it?

Yesterday was my last and final chemo treatment. I have been trying to figure out all day exactly how I feel and wondering why it is so hard.

Yes, I am glad that this will be over, but I am afraid to really believe that it is over. Dr. Greer has told me that the profile for people with my condition, CLL with a transformation to a larger cancer, not just Richter's but any larger cancer, have a strong history of recurrence. I am atypical, a clear advantage to defying statistics. Most important, I have my hovering prayer circle.

The good news is that Dr. Greer felt we could eliminate the most toxic drug, Adriamycin, for the last two chemo sessions. I responded remarkably well to the first four chemos and all visible signs of the Richter's cancer were gone after the second month, so he felt that eliminating the one drug, the most lethal, was justified. The difference without the Adriamycin (that I have recently been told is referred to as "the red devil") is huge. I have felt no nausea and am able to lead an almost normal life after the first few days.

I've spent a fair number of hours wondering how I feel about going back to my former life and what will happen next month when the effects of this chemo will subside.

The doctor has told me that they can remove the port. Some people choose to leave it in for six months or a year, just in case. To remove it is a sign of optimistic thinking. I will see Dr. Greer every month for a while; the port will be central to our dialogue.

Hugs, Sigourney

My mailbox is full by the afternoon.
Barbara writes:

Am so glad you have finally had the last treatment and I will keep my fingers crossed that the bit of hair you now have doesn't fall out. If they left out one of the most wicked drugs, maybe it won't.

We are looking forward to more boat and more family partying next summer, hopefully with all the grandchildren.

Ken writes:

Now here is my question: Did you rub "sea air, pure Spanish olive oil, Manchego cheese, fresh vegetables from the

Sunday market, and the Mediterranean sun" into your scalp? And if so, no wonder your hair didn't fall out!

Sandra writes:

How can you not focus on your hair? If I had a millimeter of anything on my head that was remotely close to hair follicles, I would probably sleep standing up and not wash them!

I will confess that I will miss your creativity with your clothes and shoes and scarves! I love seeing you put together.

I for one think that you have already ministered to many with your honesty and candor. You have set a lovely precedent for anyone facing the dread of the "C" word . . . I for one would love for you to continue your dialogue and share thoughts thru a perspective you once did not have . . . sort of a rebirth if you will. Don't stop writing please. I will have withdrawal!!!!!

Mary writes:

I want you to know how I pore over these updates and laugh and cry and am grateful for all of my blessings, not the least of which is wonderful friends. I am inspired by your courage and grace. I consider myself hugely blessed by your friendship. You are at the top of my prayer list each morning.

Carole H. writes that, as a Latin teacher, she asks her eighth graders to write their own epitaph after translating Virgil so they will think about what it means to be a human being. One made her year by writing that Carole had "taught her not to let her life slip by." Then, she goes on to thank me for my writing and:

Allowing the reader to be present with you. You have written without pretense and laid aside all vulnerability . . . a huge gift to your reader.

And another Barbara, a cancer survivor herself, thanks me for the:

OFFER OF HOPE AND GUIDANCE THROUGH YOUR HEART, EXPERIENCE, AND THE WORDS TO THE MANY STILL TO FALL PREY TO THIS ILLNESS, TO THOSE WHO ARE RECOVERING, AND TO THOSE WHO HAVE SURVIVED.

Kate assures me:

YOUR NOTES ARE GIFTS IN THEMSELVES.

And Donna adds that:

BEING GIVEN YOUR LIFE BACK ADDS SUCH A TREMENDOUS OPPORTUNITY AND RESPONSIBILITY . . . WHERE DO YOU GO FROM HERE?

Charlotte writes that:

YOU CANNOT BE TOO RICH, TOO THIN, OR HAVE TOO MANY PEOPLE PRAYING FOR YOU.

Back on the prayer list, I once again feel the comfort of those multiple prayers. I start taking the 100 mg of prednisone and have lots of time to reflect as I am up all night. I am wired. It is the worst effect yet from the stupid chemo sessions. I am glad I had been given the wrong dosage. If I ever need another round, Dr. Greer and I will have a major discussion about the dosages of prednisone. I remember Becky telling me she cleaned the kitchen-tile grout at 2:00 AM with a toothbrush after a dose of steroids, and now I understand.

I have a powerful moment at church in late November. A member whom I do not know well approaches me and asks if he could speak with me. He has just been diagnosed with a life-threatening illness, not cancer. He admires the way I handled my own illness, yet he is fearful about who he should tell about his and of being on the prayer list. I am sympathetic. I know Jim is far more reluctant to talk about his illness than I am and would never go on any public prayer list. I remind my friend that we would not be having this conversation if I had not been on the prayer list and that the circle of Christ Church family is a powerful tool of healing. We talk on, but I feel as if I haven't said enough to help.

I awake next morning at five thinking about what I could say to help my friend, praying that God would guide me. Then I remember the beautiful bi-weekly note cards sent to me by this friend and his wife with a simple sentence saying I was in their prayers. I remember thanking them after church one Sunday.

I go to the keyboard and compose a message to my friend, reminding him about the healing power of so many notes from so many friends, but telling him that they were the only couple who sent me a card saying they were thinking about me and praying for me every several weeks. There was power in those short messages that kept coming, week after week, each card more beautiful than the last with pictures of birds and flowers. If I hadn't been on the prayer list at church, those bi-weekly gifts would never have been in my mailbox.

I tell my friend I did not volunteer for the prayer list. Someone else had called and put me on. When he was ready, I would be honored to make that call for him. My friend e-mails back to tell me he cried when he read my e-mail.

I am still waiting for that call.

As I move away from chemo and talk about writing my book more than I do about my illness, people ask about my discipline for writing. And I answer, "No discipline is necessary. I can't stop." In the past, there were countless times when I didn't write for months, when the words just weren't there. But since my first day of diagnosis, I am writing or thinking about something else I need to write to clarify the last thought. I think about my audience, who I might help, and part of me realizes that it doesn't matter. Even if, as the Russians say, "I am writing for the drawer," I just have to keep writing. The writing has taken prominence over the recovery, and I have another encounter with coincidence.

I run into my journalist friend, Beth, standing in line at Bread & Company, our neighborhood deli, and we have an amazing conversation—apparently amazing for both of us. I have always admired Beth as a person and as a writer. We sit on a board together and our friendship has grown, but she would never have known about my writing if she had not been on the "Patient Siggy" list. She is encouraging about my writing in the e-mails, so I share with her an update on my book. I tell her that my literary agent advised me to find an editor or writing coach to help me create a complete and polished work if I hoped to be published. At the time I have no idea that Beth has left her last job and is searching, or that she has a background in editing. I am just playing catch-up.

The next day I receive an exciting e-mail:

AFTER TALKING TO YOU AT BREAD & COMPANY, MY PRAYER WAS THAT GOD WOULD TELL YOU WHAT YOU NEEDED TO KNOW. I OFTEN FORGET HOW SIMPLE AND POWERFUL THIS IS, AS I AM SO PRONE TO TRY AND MUSCLE THROUGH DILEMMAS ON MY OWN. I BELIEVE HE DID JUST THAT FOR YOU.

I CAN'T TELL YOU WHAT A STUNNING CONVERSATION THAT WAS FOR ME. I HAVE BEEN STRUGGLING FOR MONTHS IN SEARCH OF SOME CAREER DIRECTION THAT INSPIRES ME. FROM OUR CONVERSATION, I PICKED UP NOT ONE, BUT TWO NUGGETS—PERSONAL ESSAYS AND WRITING COACHES. IT ABSOLUTELY BLEW ME AWAY. WHETHER YOU KNEW IT OR NOT, IT WAS AN ANSWERED PRAYER FOR ME—AND CERTAINLY NO COINCIDENCE.

I WILL CONTINUE TO PRAY FOR YOU AND SURROUND YOU WITH ANGELS DURING THESE TREATMENTS. IF THERE IS ANYTHING I CAN DO FOR YOU, I'M HERE. THANKS FOR SHARING.

Beth and I have another lunch together the next week and she signs on for the task of being my editor. I couldn't have a better one.

As I work through draft seventeen (or is it twenty-seven?) of my story, I want to go back and edit the mid-October e-mail and confirm that I didn't lose my hair again. It didn't grow either. It just kind of hung in there at the same length for the last two months of treatment, and only after the chemicals receded by mid-November, did it start to grow at a snail's pace. In mid-December, it seemed to pick up speed. I want to add to the e-mail that the "fur" hair is not like my cat's hair, which is thick and strong. Mine is mole fur. But I have already sent the e-mail out into cyberspace and received responses. It's too late to edit.

Saying Adiós to the Port

*O*n the morning of the first Wednesday in December, I am to have my port removed. Jim was going to take me, but he has a persistent infection that will not respond to any of three antibiotics. He is going to have a procedure as well.

I'm not sure how I feel about Jim hogging my day for being a "patient." The "cancer twins" work out the complications of dual procedures, come home for a light lunch, and then rest.

Restored from our nap, around four, Jim gets up and sets a fire in the living-room fireplace. He and I sit in front in the two chintz chairs that face each other, wondering how we survived spring of the year 2005 with such challenging medical issues for both of us. Our bond again knits tighter, weaving in the threads of illness. We reminisce, pulling up memories of our children attending our first choice in grammar schools, Ensworth, some surviving, some not; some attending Jim's alma mater for high school, Montgomery Bell Academy, some surviving, some not; but all graduating from college, all launched into life with promising careers. Two grandchildren, another son just announcing his engagement. All this history sustains us as we face the beginning of December with the Christmas tree in the corner and the sound of the fire crackling in the granite hearth. I leave long enough to grill vegetables and salmon, and bring two plates back to enjoy by the fire with continued conversation.

The next morning I hit the keyboard.

Update from Patient Siggy

December 10, 2006

Dearest Friends,

As the holidays move closer I constantly think of the many things Jim and I are grateful for this year. Ten months ago our first granddaughter, Baker, was born. Two months ago our middle son, Daniel, became engaged to a wonderful girl from Columbus, Ohio, Anne Gilliland, and they are planning a summer wedding followed by a year in New Zealand. We'll visit. Our other boys, Jamie and Matthew, are doing well with their lives. Jamie's wife, Lisa, continues to amaze me as I watch her busy life raising Baker and Jack, yet always having time to be concerned about any needs I might have as well. I watch her and wonder how I ever had the energy to raise three boys and how it all passed so quickly.

I look back on this year and cannot believe that I have been through the trauma of cancer and seven months of chemo. Last Wednesday I had one more procedure. It was a good procedure, but I still needed to go to the hospital on an empty stomach and be put to sleep. I was having my port removed. I was turning back into a normal person, a healthy person. Jim told me he could take me, drop me off, and then come back to pick me up two hours later to drive me home. I certainly didn't need anyone to sit in a waiting room while the metal and plastic device was removed from my chest. And I was glad not to have to ask any more friends to take me to any more hospitals. This would be easy, routine.

Then Jim called at noon on Tuesday. He had been to the doctor about a persistent infection. "I have to have a procedure tomorrow too. They will have to put me to sleep and I will need someone to drive me." My first [unspoken] reaction was, "Wait a minute, tomorrow is my procedure. I am the center of attention. All sympathy goes to me." My second reaction was, "Who is driving who where?" There was silence on the phone. Jim finally said, "Look, I'll be responsible for how I get to and from my procedure and you do the same."

I was talking to Susie shortly after about our bridge schedule, and she offered to drop me off and pick me up. I

WAS SET. AS IT TURNED OUT, SUSIE AND I HAD A GREAT VISIT ON BOTH ENDS AND THE PROCEDURE WAS ROUTINE. THE SAME NURSE WHO HAD BEEN THERE WHEN THE PORT WAS PUT IN TOOK MY VITAL SIGNS, AND I THOUGHT ABOUT HOW CALM I NOW WAS ABOUT HOSPITAL ROUTINES. I WAS OUT ON TIME AND SUSIE DIDN'T EVEN NEED TO PARK. PIECE OF CAKE. SHE BROUGHT ME HOME AROUND 11:30 AND JIM WAS BACK ABOUT NOON. JAMIE WAS HIS CHAUFFEUR. IN THE FRONT OF THE HOUSE, THREE MEN WITH A CHERRY PICKER WERE STRINGING CHRISTMAS LIGHTS ON THE LARGE EVERGREEN TO THE LEFT OF THE FRONT DOOR. ONE OF THE GARDENERS WAS IN THE TOP OF ONE OF THE WEEPING CRABAPPLE TREES PRUNING. THE LAWN SERVICE HAD ONE MAN IN FRONT ON A LAWN MOWER GRINDING LEAVES. HIS HELPER WAS WALKING AROUND THE HOUSE BLOWING OFF ALL THE PATIOS. JIM AND I CLOSED THE CURTAINS IN OUR DOWNSTAIRS BEDROOM AND CRAWLED INTO BED. WE LOOKED AT EACH OTHER AND STARTED TO GIGGLE. WHAT DID THEY THINK WAS GOING ON? BOTH OUR CARS WERE IN THE BACK DRIVE. THE BEDROOM CURTAINS CLOSED. NO SIGN OF LIFE.

A ROMANTIC INTERLUDE?

WE SWAPPED OPERATION ROOM STORIES OVER THE SOUNDS OF MOTORS. I WONDERED IF I WOULD BE ABLE TO GEAR UP FOR THE HOLIDAYS. BUT NOW, A WEEK LATER, JULIE HAS COME AS SHE ALWAYS DOES AND HELPED ME DECORATE THE HOUSE. THE TREE IS BURSTING WITH SANTAS AND ANGELS AND BALLS. THE TIN STAR IS ON THE TOP AND THE FINISHING TOUCHES ARE THE FIFTY GLASS ICICLES AND THE GOLD AND CRYSTAL BEADS. THE STAIRS AND THE MANTEL ARE DRAPED IN GREEN AND THE ITALIAN ANGELS WE FOUND LAST YEAR IN SICILY ARE A TRIBUTE TO MORE–IS–GOOD AT CHRISTMAS.

I HAVE NOT WRITTEN FOR A LONG TIME BECAUSE ALL MY ENERGY IS GOING INTO WRITING MY BOOK. I DON'T KNOW IF IT WILL BE PUBLISHED OR WHO WILL READ IT, BUT I HAVE LOVED THE WRITING. IT HAS KEPT ME POSITIVELY FOCUSED. I DON'T KNOW WHEN IT IS FINISHED IF I WILL EXPERIENCE THE POSTCANCER BLUES THAT PEOPLE HAVE TOLD ME CAN FOLLOW THE END OF ALL THE ATTENTION THAT IS A NATURAL PART OF CANCER TREATMENT IF YOU HAVE ANY CIRCLE OF FRIENDS AND FAMILY.

I AM CONVINCED THAT NO ONE IN THE WORLD HAS A BETTER GROUP OF FRIENDS THAN JIM AND I HAVE. THE LOVE AND SUPPORT THAT I FELT DURING MY ORDEAL, DURING ALL OF MY PROCEDURES, HAS SUSTAINED ME. I WILL NEVER LOOK AT THE WORLD IN THE SAME

WAY. IF YOU HAVE TO BE SICK, NASHVILLE IS A NURTURING PLACE TO BE. I WILL NEVER LOOK AT MY FRIENDS IN THE SAME WAY. HOW I SEE MY FRIENDS HAS TAKEN ON A NEW DIMENSION, HAS DEVELOPED A DEEPER BOND.

ONE OF THE THINGS I HAVE NOTED IN MY BOOK IS THAT A UNIQUE INTIMACY HAS DEVELOPED THROUGH MY E-MAILS AND YOUR RESPONSES. THERE IS A SPONTANEITY NOT FOUND IN A CAREFULLY HANDWRITTEN NOTE. THERE IS A DEPTH OF SHARING WE DON'T TAKE THE TIME TO PURSUE IN QUICK PHONE OR PARTY CONVERSATIONS. ONE OF YOU WROTE, "PLEASE KEEP THE E-MAILS COMING. IF I DON'T SEE ANOTHER 'PATIENT SIGGY UPDATE,' I WILL GO INTO WITHDRAWAL." I FEEL THE SAME WHEN I READ YOUR WARM RESPONSES. I GUESS I'LL JUST HAVE TO KEEP WRITING WITH UPDATES ABOUT THE BOOK. IF IT DOESN'T GET PUBLISHED, I CAN ALWAYS SEND IT OUT TO MY CONTACT LIST. YOU ARE NOW A GROUP OF ABOUT 160 PEOPLE. WOW. I EVEN HAD TO START A SECOND CONTACT LIST. AFTER ABOUT 120 NAMES, THE LIST WOULDN'T GO WHEN I PRESSED SEND. THE PEOPLE IN COMPUTERLAND MUST NOT WANT INDIVIDUALS TO BE ABLE TO CONTACT TOO MANY PEOPLE. IS THIS A PRIVACY THING?

I'M SO GLAD THAT NASHVILLE HAS SEASONS AND THAT THE WINTER ONE IS SHORT. I LOOK FORWARD TO THE HOLIDAYS AND SILLY STOCKING GIFTS. I LOOK FORWARD TO THE FIRES AND MAYBE STAYING HOME BECAUSE OF A FEW DAYS OF SNOW AND BUNDLING UP IN A COZY SWEATER. JACK CAME OVER THIS MORNING FOR HIS FIRST TASTE OF HOT CHOCOLATE AND MINIATURE MARSHMALLOWS AND A VIEWING OF THE TREE. HE GIVES ME A HUGE SMILE AND CALLS ME SIGGY, BUT AT TWO YEARS AND TEN MONTHS HE WON'T LET ME HUG HIM. DRATS. SAD FOR US BUT EXCITING FOR HIM, DANIEL IS DOING A MONTH OF HIS MEDICAL RESIDENCY IN HAWAII, AND FOR THE FIRST TIME, ONE OF OUR SONS WILL NOT BE HERE FOR THE HOLIDAYS. BEFORE I KNOW IT, FEBRUARY WILL BE HERE AND THE FIRST WEEK WILL BE BUSY WITH ALL THE ACTIVITIES OF THE ANTIQUES AND GARDEN SHOW, MY BABY. AT THE END OF THE YEAR, CONNIE AND I ARE TURNING OVER THE RUNNING OF THE ANTIQUES SIDE OF THE SHOW TO TWO CAPABLE PAST CHAIRPEOPLE, JANETTE AND BETSY. FIFTEEN YEARS IS ENOUGH. THEN IT WILL BE MARCH AND THE GARDEN WILL START TO COME ALIVE AGAIN AND THE PEONIES WILL EMERGE, PINK AND SPIDERY BEFORE THEY CHANGE COMPLETELY.

I WISH ALL OF YOU A JOYOUS HOLIDAY SEASON. I HOPE YOU
WILL BE WITH FAMILY AND I HOPE YOU SEE THE DELIGHT ON
THE FACE OF A CHILD WHO STILL BELIEVES IN SANTA. I CAN
NEVER THANK YOU ENOUGH FOR ALL THAT YOU HAVE DONE FOR
ME THIS YEAR. BUT ONE OTHER CANCER PATIENT NOTED THAT
THIS IS A TIME TO JUST ACCEPT THE GIFTS AND NOT WORRY
ABOUT THE THANK YOUS. I JUST HOPE THAT I WILL BE MORE
ATTENTIVE TO THE NEXT FRIEND WHO NEEDS THE NURTURING
YOU HAVE GIVEN ME. I HOPE I HAVE LEARNED THE LESSON OF
PASSING IT ON.

OH, I ALMOST FORGOT: HAIR UPDATE. MY HAIR NOW COVERS
MY HEAD. IT'S ABOUT HALF AN INCH LONG. GOOD NEWS, THERE'S
VERY LITTLE GREY. PEOPLE SAY IT'S CUTE. I FEEL RIDICULOUS. IF I
WERE THIRTY AND SLIM, I THINK IT COULD BE EDGY. I SAW
PEOPLE ON THE STREET ON MY LAST VISIT TO NEW YORK WHO
WORE THIS LOOK DELIBERATELY. IT IS GROWING. IT'S BEGINNING
TO REACH MY EARS. BEFORE YOU KNOW IT I'LL NEED A TRIM. I
THOUGHT I COULD PASTE A NICE, RED BOW ON TOP FOR THE
HOLIDAYS. MAYBE NOT.

HUGS, SIGOURNEY

Within a few days the inbox is full: fifty, then seventy-five
messages. The e-mail responses coat my holiday stress with a lotion
of calm. Most are short: "YOU GO GIRL." "THANKS FOR THE UPDATE." "YOU ARE
ON MY PRAYER LIST." But others go into long paragraphs of reflection. All
are welcome and healing. My e-mails seem to be a catalyst to those
who love to write. I notice the messages encourage others to put
their own feelings into words. I have created a huge file to save the
most meaningful, longer messages. So far I have a file of two-hundred
fifty e-mail replies. Some are from close friends who follow my every
move, but others are from people at church and in the community I
barely knew before my odyssey.

Connie says:

TOUCHING AND BEAUTIFUL, I CRIED.

I don't see enough of Elizabeth, who writes:

WE ARE BLESSED THAT IN EACH OF OUR OWN WAYS (AS SMALL AS THEY MAY BE) WE WILL HAVE MUCH MORE OF YOU IN THE FUTURE . . . OUR PRAYERS HAVE BEEN ANSWERED.

And Mary Ann adds:

I FEEL AS THOUGH I'VE GOTTEN A PEEK INSIDE YOUR SOUL FROM BEING ONE OF THE RECIPIENTS OF YOUR HEALTH AND HAPPINESS UPDATES. IT'S BEEN A PRIVILEGE!

And Carole says:

THANK YOU FOR SEARCHING YOUR SOUL, YOUR FEARS, AND SHARING WITH US.

And Anne T. writes:

IT IS HARD FOR ME TO COMPREHEND THAT THIS TIME A YEAR AGO YOU WERE COMPLETELY UNAWARE OF THE CANCER AND NOT SPENDING ANY TIME IN THE CHAIR HOOKED UP TO THE TUBES. IT IS ALSO STRANGE FOR ME TO SAY I FEEL I WAS BLESSED BY YOUR ILLNESS, TO BE PART OF SUCH ABUNDANT CARING, COURAGE, AND STRENGTH—TO FEEL THE SPIRITUAL DIMENSION SO PALPABLY NEARBY.

Carole H. writes:

. . . THE BEST PART IS THE REFLECTION ON WHERE YOU WILL GO NOW. IT IS THOUGHT PROVOKING, NOT JUST FOR THE PATIENTS WHO HAVE CANCER OR ANY DISEASE, OR TRIBULATION, BUT FOR ALL OF US WHO NEED TO BE MORE REFLECTIVE ABOUT WHERE OUR LIVES ARE HEADING.

Now that all of my treatments are behind me, I look back and miss the intimate contact I had briefly felt with God during the transformation from anxiety to peace as He tossed me the life raft at the bottom of the deepest breath. How could I have let this sacred bond lapse? Why once experienced, couldn't I find the intensity again? Why didn't the experience trigger a permanent discipline of meditation? I awoke early this morning wondering when I had last consciously prayed. I recited with plodding force the words of the Lord's Prayer, my mantra to open the door. I list my family and close friends, pausing on the names of the elderly: Grandpa, Alice, Elizabeth, Eads, Dora, Caroline. I name all the people I know who have cancer or a life-threatening illness. I name the people I can remember at Christ Church who are sick. It is a rote recitation. I look back with longing, trying to exactly remember my thoughts during that sacred time, yet console myself with the knowledge that I am still at a deeper level of spiritual richness than before cancer. And I know where to find God the next time I really need to have a conversation. So maybe this is the drill, until the next crisis sparks the next epiphany and the door to the world beyond opens for a brief moment.

My priest friend, Becca, gives me insight when she explains the sacred place where I have been can only be visited. No one can dwell there. And I suspect one has to suffer deeply before being invited in the first place.

Christmas Is Coming

$\mathcal{I}$t's December. All month I am concerned I will not have the stamina to be ready for our next big event, our Christmas Eve celebration. Even though the last chemo treatment is behind me, I am still weak, tired, moving slowly. You are probably thinking, "Wasn't Mallorca enough? Let someone else do Christmas Eve." But we have hosted a Christmas Eve party for the same crowd for over thirty years. The adult children of many of our friends have been attending this event since the year they were born. I have pictures to prove it. The ritual, and believe me it is a ritual, is central to the lives of all the Cheeks and those closest to us. I feed off the adrenaline that flows from the excitement of the party being planned. Why do I groove on giving a party? One of the gifts my mother gave me was the ability to entertain with ease. I watch others stress in party mode. Maybe they are too focused on perfection. I watched my mother serve with tender, loving hands imperfect meals enjoyed by hundreds of people over the years. The relaxed atmosphere always put people at ease and resulted in a successful evening. I have attended many professionally orchestrated events and knew perfection was the least of it. I need to keep the ritual of the Christmas Eve party as the last carrot to keep me focused on the positive side of our lives as I go through the last phases of recovery. As I gently lift out of bed each morning and feel all the creaks and pains, I think, "Is this the aftermath of chemo and sick mode or is this being sixty?" I am told that exacerbated arthritis pain and being tired will last for a year after chemo. So I cling to the notion that there is an end, though not in sight, and I address the invitations to our December 24 open house. With Julie's help, the house is decorated. The first of fourteen *Amaryllis* bulbs I have planted in my collection of green McCoy pottery and placed across the three kitchen windows are opening and telling me all is well. It will be smooth sailing from here.

Then the staph infection Jim has been fighting, the staph infection that we thought would be taken care of by the procedure last week, the procedure that crashed into my procedure, will not go away. He and Dr. Roy decide he needs to spend the third week of December in the hospital for testing. I am going to cry. I feel the tears building, receding, and then building. Jim asks, "Why are you stressed? I'm the one going into the hospital." Men. I need consolation. I go into my "call-a-friend" mode. I call Jamie, leave a message; I call Nicky, leave a message; I call Carole, leave a message. Connie answers; thank you, Connie. She agrees with me about men, "Sometimes they just don't get it." Her words give me comfort as the straw floats down to break the camel's back. I am the camel. This wounded camel not only takes up residence in the middle of the living room which is already crowded because of the tree, but then moves into the kitchen, into our bedroom. I wish the camel would leave my body and turn back to wood and be satisfied as part of the hand-carved crèche scene on the chest in the front hall.

Somehow, for the next week, we manage as Jim checks into Vanderbilt and endures every possible test. Jamie brings him breakfast and the three newspapers he needs like a fix each morning. I bring lunch from Bread & Company, and return for a second visit with dinners I prepare at home. Jim needs to eat. He has lost ten pounds. Why is it that people who don't need to lose do? I negotiate the parking at Bread & Company, stand in line, and wait for the special-order sandwich he has requested, negotiate the parking at Vanderbilt, negotiate the rabbit warren of corridors in the cavernous Vanderbilt Medical Center facility from the parking below Medical Center East to the round tower in Medical Center North. At least I know the shortcuts. I am in control, moving down the antiseptic hallways, passing people in tunics with ridiculous animals and plants and nametags with pins and buttons and stickers, usually turned around so you can't read the name. (What happened to those starched white uniforms, pointy hats, and white stockings?) I arrive at Jim's green—not a Christmas green—hospital room and think about all the Christmas chores that need to be done. When I leave the hospital to do those things that need doing, I feel guilty that I'm not with Jim. Christmas and hospitals don't mix. And I know for sure that it is easier being the patient. I send warm Christmas greetings to all caregivers. You are undervalued, underappreciated. I applaud you. Every hour you can spend in the role without being pissed off is a prayer.

The Christmas to-do list has been cut to the bone. Our mailbox is stuffed with an absurd number of catalogues for the month of November and December. I think, "This is ridiculous," but it beats going to the mall, so I order stuff and watch the boxes arrive at the front door. I know I have just fed the system, and there will be more catalogues next month, next year. I slice through the plastic tape, open the stiff cardboard, sift through the Styrofoam peanuts and paper wrappings, and then drag the boxes and stuffing out to the trash. Such a waste, such an environmental nightmare, but it's Christmas and I don't have time to dispose of all the debris at the recycle dump. Bad, bad, but my list is checked off. Matthew will be happy with money; I can order something online for Daniel and

Anne from their newly established bridal registry; and we have ordered stuff for the grandbabies and Grandpa. I have cashmere sweaters for Jamie and Lisa. Jim and I will find something we both will enjoy together . . . later. Lisa and I even manage to buy, wrap, and deliver gifts for a Christmas-angel family from St. Luke's, the community center supported by Episcopal churches around Nashville.

Jim is in the hospital a full week before his infection is identified and zapped just in time to get home before Christmas Eve. Our health will be our Christmas present to each other.

It's 4:00 PM, December 24. Nicky has helped me finish everything that could possibly be finished for tonight. Silver platters, plates, and bowls wait on the table for the smoked turkey, country ham, spiced beef round, hot spinach oyster dip, hot crusted brie with almonds and dried cranberries, smoked salmon with chopped onions, capers, and of course, the wheel of Stilton cheese. I have had thirty-five years to perfect the menu, and it stays pretty much the same, year after year, another salute to ritual and tradition.

Before guests arrive, I have two hours to sit by the fireplace in the living room and look at the tree in the corner. I squint my eyes and see the hundreds of tiny white lights, the dozens of glass icicles at the end of the limbs. Outside the front window, I see the tree by the front door which I have had strung professionally for the first time with thousands of lights wrapped around each branch and down the trunk to the ground. The cat jumps up in my lap and kneads her paws into my stomach, purring. In a few hours, the house will be filled with most of the people we treasure. But the stress of having everything ready and in order increases with each year. Again I wonder if it is age or illness—probably both. I need to just relax in the decorated house with presents wrapped. I need to breathe in Christmas cheer. Everything is done. The CDs are loaded in the player. Five years ago, we added a tent to the gallery off the living room to expand the gathering space. Nicky and I have strung the twinkle lights in the boxwood hedge under the tent, and the bar table is assembled with the red-plaid tablecloth I made a million years ago. Freddy, who oversees all of our parties, will organize the bar. My diminished energy is not the only thing that has changed about Christmas Eve. It seems like only a few years ago (but I know it is longer) when I wondered why there were so many more people. Then I realized that our children were grown now and in the living room with us instead of in the playroom watching Disney movies. Now the children of our children come and sit in the playroom and watch *The Polar Express* instead of *Rudolph the Red-Nosed Reindeer*. Now the "young adults" are in their thirties instead of their twenties, and five of the daughters of close friends are about three months pregnant: Lindsey, Farrell, Craig, Lisa, and Holly. God willing, five more babies will be passed around and admired next Christmas Eve. The best part of the tradition is that all the grown children who have moved away look forward to Christmas Eve at the Cheeks' because that is where they catch up with all the people they know, but don't have time to call for lunch over the short holiday break.

This year, the last of our friends depart about 11:00 PM, and I leave Matthew with a few of his friends still catching up in the living room and go to bed. Like the birthday in Mallorca, there was something magical about the atmosphere of this year's celebration, an added joy that we are all still here and that the Cheeks are well and up for the continued tradition that is so much a part of all our lives.

Christmas Day is always informal and easy and all about the children. Jim and I wake up late, and Grandpa, who has spent the night, and Matthew come down around nine-thirty. We read and relax and wait for Jamie and his family to arrive about noon after spending the morning with Lisa's family. Jack's eyes are as big as the headlights on the red convertible car he can sit in and drive that is under the tree. "Is that for Jack?" he asks, as he climbs onboard. Within five minutes he has figured out how to push the pedal and lever on the steering wheel to make the car go back and forth, back and forth in the gallery, and he keeps pushing through his nap time and into the evening. I take a picture of Jim and Jamie and Matthew all lying on the floor in the gallery, hoping Jack will imitate them and take a short nap. He would have none of it. He is still up at 5:00 PM when we sit down to another feast, rack of lamb and Christmas crackers. The English paper funnels are wrapped in bright foil paper with a paper straw at the end that pulls open with a cracking sound to reveal a funny gag favor, a dumb riddle, and a crepe-paper hat that everyone thinks is funny after one glass of champagne. After another glass, all guilt disappears before the rich, chocolate soufflé mounded with whipped cream hits the table.

A New Year and A New Me

⚭

$\mathscr{I}$n the middle of January, I go back to Dr. Greer for a routine check-up and "all-clear" report. I have only one concern. The bug bites are back. They just reappeared one day. The bites that I can't prove but am sure came from a flea on the cat, the three bites on the left and the one on the right, are back in exactly the same place they were, starting last February, almost a year ago. They are back, and back with a vengeance, and they itch. The four bites from last year have taken up permanent residence on my neck, like mini watchdogs. The application of various versions of cortisone creams and salves is endless. Dr. Roy is puzzled. Dr. Greer is puzzled. I am trying not to scratch. We are going to do a needle biopsy in a few weeks, the same day they do a six-month-later routine PET scan and CAT scan. Six months? It couldn't be six months since the all-important PET scan in July. I count on my fingers. Yeah, it's six months.

Would I go back if I could? Never. The place I am now is too rich. I love the writing, the occasional touch with God, the constant embrace of friends, the deeper connections with hundreds of them. Coleman said, "You are a different person now." I like the enriched empathy, the deeply carved core of this new person. And are you ready for this one? I am beginning to like my hair. Someone who would never have worn short hair is beginning to groove on the "cancer cut." As my cancer survivor friend Harriet calls it, "My $65,000 haircut." Everyone says I look ten years younger. Jim loves it. "How can such short hair look good on a woman?" I ask. "I think women of a certain age just look better with short hair." I think of the few women over sixty with hair longer than their shoulders, and I know he is right. And I used to spend twenty minutes on my hair. Now I shower, towel dry, spray a little gel, fluff with my fingers to coax the little curls on the side and top into an upward thrust, and I'm done. Two minutes, max.

Connie and I go on a local talk show to pitch the Antiques and Garden Show, our favorite charity. Before the spot, I visit with our host and old friend, May Dean. She had cancer ten years ago and we talk about how she kept her hair short as well. "I used to go to the hairdresser two times a week with a very fixed do," she tells me. "I'd never go back." I tell May Dean I want to talk about my shorter-than-short hair. On the air, May Dean reminds the audience she was a cancer survivor and then turns to me. "I love my cancer cut," I say, "I would never have cut my hair short and now I love it. And surprisingly, the men think it's sexy. Go figure. This has become a cancer perk." I feel empowered passing this tidbit into TV land. Connie and I also manage to promote the show, of course.

As I look back, the way I chose to deal with my illness was to not listen to other people's war stories, to not linger on some other hospital that might have done a better job in a better city, to not seek out anyone who Mary Jane and Carole describe as "crepe hangers," those who dig into the worst part of illness and linger there, focused on the worst pain, sure that the worst diagnosis will materialize. I need to keep my glass half full, the legacy of my father whose optimism inspired me. From where does the optimism gene emerge? Even as opposite personality types, Jim and I both share this trait. Why?

Janet gave me this story the other day. Perhaps wisdom from another culture hits the mark. A Cherokee grandfather is teaching his grandson about life. "A fight is going on inside me," he tells the boy. "It is a terrible fight between two wolves. One is evil—he is anger, envy, sorrow, regret, greed, arrogance, self-pity, guilt, resentment, inferiority, lies, false pride, superiority, and ego."

He continues, "The other wolf is good—he is joy, peace, love, hope, serenity, humility, kindness, benevolence, empathy, generosity, truth, compassion, and faith.

"The same fight is going on in you and inside every other person."

The grandson thinks a minute and then asks, "Which wolf wins?"

The old Cherokee replies, "The one you feed."

I went to Roy in December for my first official physical. I am now trying to be responsible about my health. We talked about fighting illness in a positive way. His experience is that people draw from their strength, whatever that may be. For Jim it is sports, staying fit, keeping up his pace at work.

Thanks to the journey over the last ten months I have learned what my strengths are as well. Looking back, one of my strengths is entertaining: the Garden Conservancy dinner, the once-in-a-lifetime birthday bash, the annual Christmas Eve celebration. I certainly wasn't willing to let go of any of them as was suggested by many. Each of them provided a focus outside my treatments, a goal on the horizon that I anticipated with pleasure.

One of my strengths is a willingness to embrace community. After my first month of terror, I turned to my faith, my friends at Christ Church, my e-mail team, my family and closest friends who are also my family. I was never alone, and I will never be the same. When the threat of death visits again, I hope I will be eighty. But if it is sooner, I will cope. I have learned the fear of death is only in the unknowing. I wake up some mornings remembering a recurring dream, or rather a layer of dreams, about the cancer returning. I awake knowing the dream closest to the surface is just a dream, but the one underneath it seems real. Then I clear a few more sleep cobwebs to confirm that the one underneath, the one deeper in my unconscious, is a dream as well. I hope it will continue to be a dream, but the possibility of transformation to reality is constantly with me. I'm surprised, but it doesn't frighten me. My writing tells me that I will handle the next round. After all, I was OK with the dress rehearsal.

One of my strengths is writing. The painful parts become bearable for me through writing. At the keyboard I can focus on the first peony opening in our Nashville garden; the morning birds' calls in the treetop room in Monteagle; Jim's toast on the wall of El Barco in Mallorca; Baker in the hand-stitched, peach, batiste dress I finished for her to wear Christmas Eve—the same one I started thirty-five years ago when one of our three boys was going to be a girl. If my words help others find deeper meaning in the fight against cancer, how honored I would be.

I choose to use positive moments in my life as carrots instead of participating in a cancer support group, instead of listening to many I-had-cancer-too stories. Dr. John told me many people experience muscle aches from the white-blood booster shot chemo patients receive twenty-four hours after the chemo. "Well," I said, "Nobody told me, so I missed that one." Maybe others see as a horse with blinders on, but with blinders on, the horse sees only what is necessary to stay the course. I knew that was all I could handle at the beginning, staying the course.

Another friend, Jane, who has MS, responded to my December e-mail: "I am thrilled to read about your journey, which you describe so well and with great insight. Still wish you and I did not have to take this arduous journey . . . you and I do not get to choose the itinerary, it seems!"

I have been back to the dermatologist at Vanderbilt who specializes in cancer patients to biopsy one of my bug bites. The test result proves the bumps on my neck that became infected and led to an early diagnosis of my disease were indeed just bug bites. My immune system does not know how to respond because of the CLL, and the little soldiers that should fight and heal this affliction are confused or blocked. On the return visit, the doctor gives me cortisone shots on each bite to finally make them go away, after ONE year. What a weird symptom, itchy lumps for a year. Hopefully this first symptom will become the last.

It is now February, and it has snowed. They predicted inches, but as often happens in Nashville, the reality is a light frosting on the grass and flower beds. I go to the kitchen bookshelf where I have stored the envelope containing the poppy pods I stole on the way home from chemo one. Most of the seeds have fallen out of the pods and rest in the bottom fold of the envelope, smaller than grains of sand. I go out to the crescent-shaped bed off our bedroom, pinch a selection of miniscule dots, and sprinkle black seeds over white snow.

Another spring is almost here. It is a year from the first signs of illness. Reflecting back I find more blessings than sorrow. My life has been enriched more than diminished by the experience. I am a different person and I like the new me. I like the deepening friendships nurtured by e-mail messaging. No, I cannot choose my itinerary, but I can choose how to navigate the path. My heart full of gratitude, I sit down for one more contact with cyberspace.

UPDATE FROM UNPATIENT SIGGY
END OF FEBRUARY
DEAREST FRIENDS,

I LOOK BACK ON THE LAST YEAR, AND THINK BEING DIAGNOSED WITH CANCER IS SCARY, HORRIBLE, LIFE-CHANGING. BUT RISING FROM THE HORROR, SO MUCH RICHNESS HAS COME FROM THIS

JOURNEY, THE GIFT OF A DEEPENING FAITH, THE GIFT OF AN INCREDIBLE NUMBER OF FRIENDS WHO HAVE OVERWHELMED ME WITH NOTES AND FLOWERS AND FOOD AND VISITS AND SHARED STORIES, THE GIFT OF EXPERIENCING THE POWER OF PRAYER AND EMBRACING THE CONSTANT LOVE OF PEOPLE WHO WERE LINED UP, YES LITERALLY LINED UP, TO BRING DINNER, TAKE ME TO CHEMO, COME BY FOR THE VISIT WE'D BEEN TALKING ABOUT AND IS FINALLY REALIZED.

DO I JUST GO BACK TO LIFE AS USUAL AFTER THIS TRANSFORMATION? CAN I FIND MORE MEANING IN THE YEARS AHEAD? THERE MUST BE A WAY I CAN GIVE SOME OF THIS BACK. SO MANY SUFFERERS LACK THE SUPPORT TEAM I HAVE ENJOYED. BUT I DON'T THINK MY SKILLS INCLUDE REGULARLY HOLDING THE HAND OF SICK STRANGERS.

I DO KNOW THAT I WILL SPEND MORE TIME WITH MY FRIENDS, HAVE MORE COMPASSION WHEN SOMEONE IS SICK, ENJOY MY FAMILY, MY GRANDCHILDREN. I WILL ENJOY THE TURNED YELLOW TREES THIS FALL, THE EARLIEST FLAKES OF SNOW THIS WINTER. I ALREADY DREAM ABOUT THE FIRST PEONY THAT WILL OPEN IN MY GARDEN, SOMETIME IN LATE APRIL OR EARLY MAY. I WILL PICK IT, BRING IT INSIDE, PUT IT IN MY GREEN VASE ON THE GREEN, PAINTED CHEST IN MY BEDROOM AND THINK ABOUT THIS PAST APRIL, WHEN MY ODYSSEY BEGAN. I WILL CIRCLE THE GARDEN EACH AFTERNOON, FOCUSED ON EACH NEW PEONY OPENING, REMEMBERING THIS PAST APRIL AND BEING MINDFUL OF WHERE EACH SENSUOUS WHITE, BLUSH-PINK OR BUTTER-YELLOW BLOOM IS LEADING ME NOW.

HUGS, SIGOURNEY

Writing Workshop

thought my story was finished and life was back to a comfortable routine. I was so wrong. Thank God I found a new focus before moving into lazy summer mode. The new gear started with a call from my priest friend, Becca. She sent me down a path into unfamiliar territory with surprising results. She opened a door into a ministry of healing and showed me a way to use writing to heal others.

A cause I feel strongly about is Magdalene House, a halfway house in Nashville for women who have been on the street. Becca is the genius behind this success story. The community she has created is relatively small: three houses for four women each and another for eight, but the impact is large. Eighty-five percent of the women move on to full, productive lives. As I struggle with my own challenges of health and spiritual quests, I feel a connection to these women and their plight. I feel a passion to help.

Anyone in Becca's orbit is affected by her gift of unconditional love. In the atmosphere she creates, the women of Magdalene and the women in the community who help them, meld to form unusual friendships and become allies and compatriots. Both groups benefit from the unique experience.

Several months ago, Becca announced an interest from her publisher in the publishing of the handbook on how Magdalene House is run. "Who would like to help with this project?" I was one of several who raised a hand.

The book is currently written in the voice of Becca and her staff. The publisher wanted it to be in the voices of the women in recovery. Becca called several weeks later and asked if I would lead a writing workshop for the women and try to find their voices. A retreat had been planned for Memorial Day weekend at St. Mary's Retreat Center on Monteagle Mountain. Could I come and lead a two-hour workshop that Friday?

I calculate. I plan to spend Memorial Day weekend with my family at our place in Ponte Vedra, Florida. There are four flights a day from nearby Jacksonville to Nashville, one in the early morning and another in the evening. I know, somehow, I need to say, "Absolutely." I have never given a workshop to anyone on anything, but I could try. And if I succeeded, this new use of the written word could enhance my life. After all, cathartic writing is my specialty. I instinctively know these women have unique stories to tell, and in the right atmosphere, journaling could help release them. I remember lessons on writing learned from writing gurus Anne Lamont and Natalie Goldberg, and I prepare some notes about how to proceed with a workshop and send a copy to Becca. This would be a fly-by-the-seat-of-the-pants operation, but it could work.

The following Friday morning I wake up at the beach at 5:30, drive to the airport to arrive at 6:30. The flight leaves at 7:15 and arrives in Nashville at 7:40, central time. The drive from the airport to Monteagle takes an hour, and St. Mary's Retreat Center is another twenty minutes away.

I arrive about 9:30 AM, with half an hour to spare before the beginning of my two-hour workshop. I meet the women coming inside after a meditation exercise outside, looking down the mountain from the edge of the retreat center. The day is warm, the air clear, and the women are relaxed in the quiet beauty of the space. The thirty women range in age from about twenty to fifty-five, half white, half black. They walk towards me in two lines, arms entwined. After years shared on the street, they bond like sisters on holiday.

We go inside and gather in a room with a circle of chairs. I start with a short prayer. I apologize for reading but explain this is a new experience for me. We hold hands. I have to keep one free for my prayer:

> Dear Lord,
>
> Thank You for giving me the gift of understanding for the first time at age sixty the real meaning of prayer. With last year's glimpse into the possibility of my life being over because of the threat of a bad cancer, people were saying prayers for me instead of the other way around, and for the first time, I confronted the exact meaning of prayer.
>
> Thank You for this insight: when a group of us are gathered together in Your name, You are with us in a special way and this is a prayer.
>
> Thank You for helping me see that when I write and ask You to sit on my shoulder, my words stay honest and I am able to dig deep into my heart where secrets lie in hidden spaces and then my words turn into a prayer.
>
> Help all of us here today to be focused and to do soulful work in describing the healing work of our life at Magdalene so that the pains and joys of our experience can be passed on. Let our voices help other pilgrims on the road. Let our words turn into a prayer.
> Amen.

I tell the women about my experience with meditation and deep breathing and connecting with God and my spiritual core. I share the story about being sick and riddled with anxiety and fear for the first month of my illness, thinking I might die, thinking this could be it. I explain my exercise: breath deeply into your diaphragm, breath out, slowly—deeper. Invite Jesus in. I tell them I invited the whole family in, God the Father; Jesus; Sophia, the spirit, my feminine face of God; and the Blessed Virgin; and suddenly my anxiety was gone. I was at peace, totally calm. I hope sharing my story and exercise will help the ladies be in the right place to start writing.

The thirty women sit in a large circle around the circumference of the meeting room. I pass out writing paper I found at a discount store called Fred's on the way up the mountain. The paper is covered with images of pale-pink angels and leaves from mountain trees. Is it a coincidence finding thirty coordinating writing pads in a small store? I pass out colored pens, enough for each person to have several colors.

Reading through the Magdalene handbook a few weeks earlier, I jotted down key phrases to sum up the essence of the journey. I tell the women, "I will give you one phrase at a time. Try first to find a peaceful place. Ask God to sit on your shoulder. Don't think in grand, lofty concepts. Keep the writing in a positive voice. Give me small details: the temperature of the room, the time of day, the smells in the air, who is next to you, how the chair you are sitting in feels, if your shoes hurt. Make me feel the moment. (My favorite author on writing, Anne Lamont, calls this a "shitty first draft.") I say, "You have ten minutes to write on each topic."

I start with the topic "a trip to the dentist or a doctor's visit." (I have read that many of the women have never been to the doctor until entering the program.) In the room, you could have heard a pin drop, feel the sacred quality to the air, sense the power of concentration and hard work being accomplished. I ask one of the women to be a time-keeper. Hope volunteers and calls out at the end of ten minutes.

We continue with several topics, for example, "Small changes make all the difference; healing happens slowly. When did you feel a change?", "Describe the sisterhood of the circle. How does it feel?" and "Describe the walk down Dickerson Road looking for a customer." I want to uncover poignant moments and trigger gut-wrenching responses.

After an hour we take a break and I say to Becca, "I think some of the women would like to read one of their pieces." She replies, "Absolutely." After the break, I ask if anyone wants to read. Surely three or four would be brave. We sit through a moment of silence, and then one of the ladies raises her hand. Her voice is hesitant at first, but she soon is in the groove. The words are beautiful and heartbreaking.

At the doctor she was told that an HIV test was negative:

> While I was rejoicing about that, the doctor slid in on me I have hepatitis C. My face turned into a frown of sadness. After taking this news in, I immediately shut down and didn't want to talk to anyone. Me, me, poor me.
>
> Nobody will understand, nobody cares.
>
> In reality I know if I let someone know, they will care. Wow, I told the truth to my paper and I haven't shared this with all my Magdalene sisters because of what they might think of me. I know I really know better.

At the end, everyone applauds through tears for the courage she demonstrates by letting the pad and pen unlock the secrets in her heart. Many of the group give the reader a supportive hug and hand her the roll of toilet tissue being passed around instead of Kleenex.

Another woman caught the beauty of Becca:

> I sat here and didn't feel anything on our title of the writing assignment. But as I sit here quietly, enjoying the peace, Becca gets up and walks over to Tracy and starts braiding her hair. That is when I felt something and began to write. Of course the feeling was love and I am amazed

as I look at her go from Tracy's hair to Kathy, judging no
one and being one of us, the comfort of being around her.
So soothing inside of the intimidation that enters my heart.

Another participant reads her piece, and then another, and then
another. The next hour is filled with the voices of all thirty women,
each and every one reading one of her pieces. I take that back. One
woman has a scribe. She can't read or write. The volunteer scribe
reads her piece.

Each reading is rich and honest and healing, and beauty perme-
ates the words. The women are excited, empowered, and proud of
their achievements.

I stay to have lunch with the group and ask for a volunteer from
each house who is computer literate to record each essay and enter
them into a Word document. I know we will find enough fodder for
the Magdalene book to be converted into the voices of the women
in recovery. I know that we will meet again, write again. I know the
Magdalene book will be a small part of deeper work and more words
will bring us together along a path of healing.

I drive back to the Nashville airport, take the late flight back to
Jacksonville, and make the forty-minute ride back to the beach, back
to my family. I walk through the door of our place at 8:00 PM and
catch the tail end of their day in the sand.

A Wedding and More Mallorca

⁓

$\mathcal{I}$plan to meet with the women again when I return from another August in Mallorca. The beginning of the summer is filled with activities, including Anne and Daniel's wedding on the weekend of the Fourth of July. Anne and her family are from Columbus, so the wedding is at Salt Fork Lodge on a pristine lake in the largest state park in the middle of Ohio.

Our first thought is how to get from here to there with our assorted family members ranging from ages eighty-eight to under two. Can we turn a challenge into an opportunity? Our oldest son, Jamie, works in the entertainment business and frequently rents a big, luxurious tour bus for one of his musician clients. I had often passed these buses on the road and wondered what they would be like on the inside. Grandpa, Jamie, Lisa, Jack, Baker, and Lisa's mom, Nancy, are traveling with us. We decide all those airline tickets versus the cost of a bus is close to a wash, so Jamie hires the fantasy bus. Our youngest son, Matthew, and his girl-friend, Jessie, are so excited they fly from Colorado to Nashville to go with us. Thursday morning, the bus and driver are at our back door by 8:00 AM. We load luggage and all the props for the rehearsal dinner picnic, including flower pots, candles, cheerful red bandanna tablecloths, paper napkins, plates, and cutlery. We even rent a margarita machine. There is plenty of room under this sucker, so why not?

The bus has a large living area in the front with facing sofas, a TV, and a kitchen with a full-size fridge. The center of the bus has a bathroom and twelve bunks, stacked three high, with a TV screen in each. When the bus is stationary, one side of the front room pushes out three feet for added comfort. The back of the bus is another large sitting room with a wraparound sofa and a huge TV. Jamie tells us the back room is where the action happens on music tours. On our trip, it is where the guys hang out and watch an endless stream of sporting events.

We have loaded the bus with chips and dips, and cokes and beer, and the seven-hour drive goes by in a flash. The bus does not just sit idly during our four days at the park. The wedding party uses it each night for after-party parties until the wee hours. Two of Dan's friends drive all the way from Maine. They arrive on Thursday, in the middle of the night, and their reservation is not until Friday. They roll their sleeping bags out on the lawn next to the bus. All is well until the sprinkler system goes off at 5:30 AM.

Anne's family is warm and laid back, and the atmosphere of the long weekend takes on

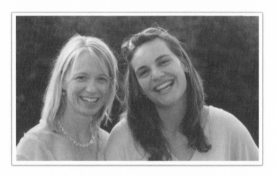

Jamie's wife, Lisa, and Matthew's girlfriend, Jessie, at pre-wedding festivities.

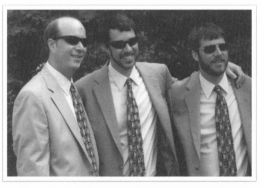

The three brothers on Daniel's wedding day. From left: Jamie, Daniel, and Matthew.

the feel of old friends gathering instead of new ones, almost like a big family reunion.

The wedding ceremony is in a lush field behind the lodge. Anne's three sisters and Dan's two brothers and cousin Nicholas make up the wedding party. For the reception, the center of each table has a different flavored, hand-baked cake decorated with wild flowers. After the toasts, people move around the room from one table to the next, sampling carrot, chocolate, and caramel cakes, and then dance hard to work off the indulgence.

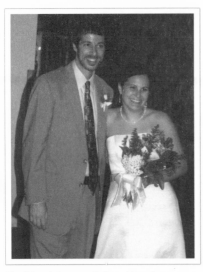

Daniel and Anne on their wedding day.

Anne reminds me of myself at her age, and I look forward to rich times ahead. How could I be so lucky with both daughters-in-law? My mother and mother-in-law have been gone for more than ten years, and I am celebrating adding women to our family of all men.

I spend the rest of the time before Mallorca finishing the last draft of my book, determined to send the final copy to my literary agent in Washington before leaving for Spain. This time I am healthy, with my snappy, new, short haircut.

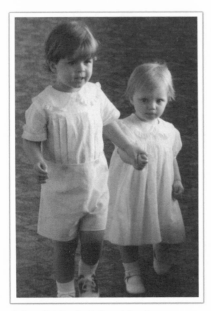

Jack and Baker in their wedding best.

I realize I haven't written to my contact group since late February. Before the trip, I fire off an update about my book instead of my illness.

UPDATE FROM UNPATIENT SIGGY
JULY 25, 2006
DEAR FRIENDS,

REMEMBER ME? AS A WELL PERSON, I DO NOT SEEM TO HAVE THE SAME DRIVE TO KEEP IN TOUCH WITH ALL OF YOU. ALL OF MY BEST INTENTIONS AND GOOD RESOLUTIONS HAVE GONE DOWN THE DRAIN. WHAT WAS I THINKING? I MISS YOU. I MISS THE PERSONAL MESSAGES THAT USED TO FILL MY INBOX ON A REGULAR BASIS. NOW MY INBOX IS FILLED WITH BOARD MEETING AGENDAS, POTTERY BARN ADS, NEW PALM SOFTWARE OPPORTUNITIES, VIACOM UPDATES. BORING.

FOR THE LAST SIX MONTHS, MY WRITING ENERGY HAS BEEN GOING INTO FINISHING MY BOOK BETWEEN TOO MANY OTHER ACTIVITIES. UNPATIENT SIGGY HAS GOTTEN RIGHT BACK INTO HER OVER-PROGRAMMED LIFE. BAD, BAD, BAD. IN JUNE WE HOSTED THE BIG SWAN BALL PATRON PARTY FOR DEAR CONNIE'S SWAN BALL, AND I REDID ALL THE STUFF YOU THINK ABOUT REDOING BUT NEVER GET AROUND TO.

MY PERSONAL FAVORITE: I HAVE AN ELECTRICIAN FROM SOUTHERN LIGHTS OVER TO REDO MY OUTDOOR LIGHTING. I TRIED TO DO IT MYSELF FIRST. I WAS AT EXPO, THE NEW DESIGN PLACE NEXT TO HOME DEPOT IN HUNDRED OAKS THAT HAS EVERY-THING—INCLUDING A HUGE SELECTION OF KITCHEN SINKS. I WAS BUYING STUFF FOR THE RENOVATION OF OUR MONTEAGLE HOUSE AND SAW A NEW OUTDOOR LIGHTING SYSTEM THAT SEEMED TO BE PRETTY REASONABLE. I BOUGHT IT AND CALLED AN ELECTRICIAN TO HELP INSTALL IT. I THOUGHT WE WOULD BE OFF AND RUNNING. IT WAS A DISASTER. THERE WERE ALL THESE COMPLICATED ISSUES ABOUT BALANCING THE RIGHT NUMBER OF AMPS ACROSS THE RIGHT WIRES. NEVERMIND. THE LIGHTS KEPT BLOWING FUSES AND EVEN WHEN THEY WERE ALL ON, THERE WAS NOT ENOUGH LIGHT IN THE GARDEN. I MADE AN SOS CALL TO OUR CONTRACTOR, IN A PANIC A WEEK BEFORE THE PATRON PARTY. HELP. HE TOLD ME ABOUT THE BEST OUTDOOR-LIGHTING GURU, JOHN SCULLY AT SOUTHERN LIGHTS. I KNEW IT WOULD BE EXPENSIVE, BUT ALL THESE MUCKITY-MUCKS WERE COMING NEXT WEEK. THEY WOULD BE ALL OVER MY

GARDEN AT NIGHT. I WAS STUCK. I WAS LUCKY JOHN HAD THE TIME TO RESCUE ME. WE BECAME BEST FRIENDS. HE HAD GREMLINS ALL OVER THE GARDEN FOR DAYS AND FIXED THE LIGHTS. THEY ARE STATE-OF-THE-ART. IN PASSING, I FOUND OUT HE HAD DONE THE SAME THING AT THE HOUSES OF TWO OTHER PATRON PARTY HOSTESSES IN VERY RECENT YEARS RIGHT BEFORE THEIR BIG NIGHTS.

IN JULY, WE HAD DANIEL AND ANNE'S WEDDING IN OHIO. IT WAS SMALL AND INTIMATE AND VERY SPECIAL. HER FAMILY IS WONDERFUL AND OURS HAS EXPANDED. ALL SPRING I DROVE UP TO MONTEAGLE ONCE A WEEK UNTIL WE FINISHED, ALMOST, THE RENOVATION OF GRANDPA'S COTTAGE IN MONTEAGLE IN TIME FOR THE OPENING OF THE SEASON THE SECOND WEEK IN JUNE. SOMEWHERE IN THE MIDDLE OF ALL THE OTHER MAJOR EVENTS, I FINISHED THE BOOK. AS I EDITED MY MANUSCRIPT OVER MANY MONTHS, I WOULD GET TO THE PARTS WHERE IT SAID, "I'LL NEVER GO BACK TO THE OVER-PROGRAMMED PERSON I USED TO BE." AND THEN I WOULD THINK, "LIAR, LIAR, PANTS ON FIRE, HYPOCRITE, PHONY BALONEY." NOW I AM GOING TO GIVE MYSELF ANOTHER SHOT AT MY BEST INTENTIONS FOR LAST YEAR. HEADING TO A QUIET AUGUST IN MALLORCA WITH FAMILY WILL HELP.

I HAVE AN ADRENALINE RUSH FROM MAILING A COPY OF *Patient Siggy: Hope and Healing in Cyberspace—an Antidote for the Isolation of Illness* TO MY AGENT, MY REAL LITERARY AGENT, IN WASHINGTON ABOUT AN HOUR AGO. THE E-MAILS FROM THE PAST YEAR OF ILLNESS AND RECOVERY ARE THE BACKBONE, THE SKELETON OF THE BOOK.

BETH HAS HELPED ME FOR THE PAST TWO MONTHS AS EDITOR. I DELETED THE WORD "THAT" 300 TIMES. I PUT PUNCTUATION INSIDE FIFTY QUOTE MARKS. I CHANGED FIFTY TO 50. WE WON'T GO INTO MY SPELLING. LOSE, LOOSE, WHAT'S THE DIFFERENCE?

SHE ASKED ME TO SUM UP WHAT THE BOOK IS ABOUT AND WHAT I HOPED TO PASS ON TO THE READER SO I GAVE IT A SHOT:

MY BOOK IS ABOUT A CONFRONTATION WITH DEATH, THE GROWTH OF AN INTIMATE DIALOGUE BETWEEN AN EVER-INCREASING NUMBER OF FRIENDS, AND THE HEALING POWER OF THE E-MAIL CHAIN THAT BECAME A SACRED CIRCLE SHARED BY ALL.

MY HOPE IS THAT THE BOOK WILL TEACH OTHERS ABOUT POWER: THE POWER OF COMMUNAL PRAYER, THE POWER OF CHOOSING A POSITIVE PATH TO FIGHT THROUGH SERIOUS ILLNESS, THE POWERFUL CATHARSIS OF SHARING THE STRUGGLE THROUGH

WRITING, AND THE POWER OF COMMUNICATING IN CYBERSPACE AS
AN ANTIDOTE FOR THE ISOLATION OF ILLNESS.

I WISH I COULD ASK FOR PRAYERS FOR THE PUBLICATION, BUT I
BELIEVE THAT THOSE NEED TO BE SAVED FOR LIFE-AND-DEATH MATTERS.
GOD IS BUSY. BUT IF YOU COULD ALL USE YOUR POSITIVE THINKING,
MAYBE, JUST MAYBE, IT WILL CROSS OVER TO PUBLICATION LAND.

I HAVE BIRTHED A BABY, NUMBER FOUR, THE OTHER ONE JIM
AND I TALKED ABOUT HAVING LONG AGO. THANK GOD WE CAME TO
OUR SENSES.

TOMORROW, TEE HEE, I WILL HAVE MESSAGES FROM SOME OF
YOU. I CAN'T WAIT.

HUGS, SIGOURNEY

Reconnecting with my support team keeps me busy for the last week of July, and then I lift off to cross the ocean. We are back in El Barco, our magical house by the sea. The days starts at dawn with the pink glow behind the marina and La Victoria Mountain on the right, outside our bedroom window. I turn over and drift back into sleep for a few more hours. Then I walk down the narrow, stone steps, curving into the back of the tower that forms the master bedroom up and the living room down, and go into the kitchen for Greek yogurt and cut-up, doughnut-shaped peaches called paraguyas. I go out to the terrace and sit and take in the panoramic sea views in front of me, sipping coffee and writing in my journal and wondering what bits will translate into words to be passed on.

A few friends who were here last summer join us again, Dana and Tom, Claudie and Doug, and we add another ten days of shared Spanish summer memories. This summer is all about relaxation and fun. A highlight is a cooking lesson in Barbara's kitchen, to make "coca," a Mallorcan pizza. Everyone is laid back and at ease with the routine, until August 17, and then my life shatters all over again. I turn upside down, sideways, tumbling.

After an afternoon excursion and lunch of grilled fish in the Port of Sollier, we return to our house. In the late afternoon, I feel

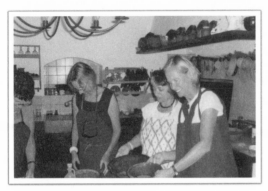

Learning to make "coca" in Barbara's kitchen.
From left: Siggy, Barbara, Claudie, and Dana.

something under my right arm. I lift my arm over my head and feel a lump. A big lump. Oh God, please no. Is this really happening? Alert. Full stop. I am crashing into another hairpin turn. I am cut off a second time from where I was going. I fear a long and challenging detour ahead. On the other hand, the lump is not as big as the last time and it's not as sore. Yet, it is there. I think of the now bi-monthly meetings with Dr. Greer and his upbeat reports after probing all the areas where lymph nodes exist in my body, and the "everything is fine" reports.

Well, everything is not fine. My hands grip the kitchen counter. How do I feel? I keep wondering. I am undecided, restless, and numb at the same time. The next morning, I feel another lump in my right groin. Shit, shit, shit. I was so sure I would be one of the lucky ones, counting year after year of remission. Hadn't they all said I was the poster child of the CHOP+R regime?

I keep lifting my arm to feel if the lump is bigger, smaller. It's the same. I remember Dr. Greer's response to the question, "Will my cancer come back?" He said, "In eighteen months to three years." I count on my fingers. It has been ten months since the last chemo. Jim suggests maybe I am supposed to count from the beginning of chemo, which would make it sixteen months. Good try Jim, but I don't think so. My sister-in-law, Barbara, suggests maybe it is just some allergic reaction. Good try Barbara, but I don't think so.

We call Dr. Roy and he doesn't feel I need to come home early, unless I am too anxious. I do a mental tally. I am shocked I do not have the anxiety I experienced with the first diagnosis. Surely this will be a lesser cancer, a more treatable cancer. Maybe I won't even need immediate treatment. I am determined to enjoy the last two weeks of the month. I need these two weeks. And surprisingly enough, for the most part, I'm OK. Some of the peace I resurrected last spring from the bottom of my diaphragm must be left over. I don't count the middle-of-the-night awakenings when the "what ifs" prompt me to read for a few hours and not think. During the day, I put the lump away in a secluded part of my brain.

With three days to go, my nephew, Alexander, comes down in the morning and tells his mother he had a dream about Aunt Siggy. I should go to his homeopathic doctor in Palma. He asks his mom, "Do you think this is just a coincidence or should I tell Aunt Siggy?"

The practice of alternative medicine is widely accepted throughout Europe. My brother and his family are huge believers in homeopathic healing. I have never given much thought to an alternative way of looking at the body and healing. I'm just aware of my brother and sister-in-law taking herbs instead of antibiotics. Barbara reports the dream to me, saying. "I don't want you to do anything that makes you uncomfortable." I tell Barbara, "Don't you remember the first paragraph of my book? I don't believe in coincidence. Let's make the appointment. Why wouldn't I try any avenue possible towards healing?" Alexander makes the call, and for twenty-four hours, he hears nothing. "Maybe the doctor, Gabriel, is away." I say, "Oh, I know we will get an appointment." I know more than coincidence is at work, and sure enough, the next day Gabriel calls. He arranges to meet me at his office, on his day off, on the last full day I will be in Mallorca.

We drive to Palma on the new motorway, around the industrial town of Inca, taking fifteen minutes off the trip. Gabriel, half-French, half-Spanish, is fifty-something, soft-spoken and approachable. With a combination of English, French, and Spanish, and Barbara helping with difficult translations, Gabriel examines my aura, the energy field surrounding a person, and my chakra points, seven major energy centers within the physical body. He uses acupressure and computer programs to help balance these energy fields. He explains a balanced body is a healthy body. My aura has shown trouble spots: my lymph-node system, my spleen, my heart, stress in my head—hello. For the next two hours, a new and complicated world opens as I am introduced to ancient, two-thousand-year-old healing practices that have been generally ignored in the United States. As I try to absorb the gist of this probing and aligning, I am thinking that with this next round of cancer, I will be proactive in exploring all possible paths to healing and health.

He gives me "Bach Flower Remedy" drops, the essence of certain flowers to take before and after each meal to help repair my damaged systems. He looks in my mouth and tells me I need to remove all my mercury fillings as soon as possible. He points to the fourth tooth on the lower left and says, "Especially that one which corresponds to your lymph-node system." I leave puzzled, yet pumped. If I must fight again, I will go on a quest to research all possible resources. I am already off with a stronger start.

I come home on August 31 to lots of Western doctors and lots of tests. Thank goodness, Dr. Roy, unlike many doctors, is a student of Chinese medicines and willing to enter into a dialogue on the possible benefits of interactive healing; yoga; breathing; sound, good nutrition; and maybe herbs and oils to compliment traditional Western medical practices.

I go to my dentist, Dr. Gary, and explain about the mercury fillings. Instead of thinking I'm nuts, he reports patients who have requested the removal of mercury. He is familiar with the careful covering of the extracted area to suck out the mercury and prevent it from entering the body during removal. He looks in my mouth. "I could do the two on the left right now." He numbs the left side and looks again. "The two on the other side are fairly small. Come back another day and I could take care of them in half an hour." A little voice comes from nowhere, "By any chance, would you have time to take them all out today?" He agrees, with no appointment! I leave with a swollen face and my jaw is sore for three days, but I am thrilled I did it, even if the change improved my chances of recovery by one-half a percent.

I call my favorite florist and send a large bouquet to his office with a thank-you note and a copy of the article on the front page of the business section of today's the *Wall Street Journal*, Tuesday, September 12, 2006, "Metal Mouth: Do You Need to Worry about the Mercury in Dental Fillings?" Another coincidence? It even has a quote from a doctor at Vanderbilt who is a specialist in mercury. I can't wait to send him an e-mail.

A phone call the next day from Dr. Greer with the results of my medical tests brings terrible news. As always I find comfort at the keyboard, giving another dimension to the facts and reaching out once again to my awesome support group.

UPDATE FROM PATIENT SIGGY—ROUND 2
SEPTEMBER 14, 2006
DEAR WONDERFUL FRIENDS,
AUGUST IN MALLORCA WAS BLISS, THE SOUNDS AND TASTES OF ANOTHER SPANISH SUMMER IN OUR HOUSE BY THE AQUA SEA, SHARED WITH FRIENDS AND FAMILY. LEISURE AMUSEMENTS

BROUGHT PEACE AND REST, AT LEAST UNTIL THE SEVENTEENTH OF THE MONTH. WE WENT OUT ON MY BROTHER KEVIN'S OLD FISHING BOAT, AND I COULD ONCE AGAIN CLIMB TO THE BOW AND DIVE INTO THE TURQUOISE WATER AND SLICK MY HAIR BACK AND KNOW ALL WAS RIGHT WITH THE WORLD. EVERY TIME I HIT THE WATER, I WOULD REMEMBER THE YEARS I HAD PLUNGED BELOW THE SURFACE, NEVER GIVING IT A THOUGHT. THE LAST SUMMER WITH NO HAIR AWOKE A REVERENCE FOR WHICH RITUALS IN LIFE ARE IMPORTANT. THE TOP FOR ME ARE FAMILY GATHERINGS, ESPECIALLY IF YOU REALLY LOVE EACH OTHER AND ARE IN THE PLACES WHERE MEMORIES ARE STACKED ON TOP OF EACH OTHER. GIVEN THE CHOICE, WE WOULD BE WITH EACH OTHER, ANYTIME, ANYPLACE. DIVING IN THAT WATER, I STAYED UNDER FOR A FEW STROKES AND ABSORBED THE POWER OF EACH PLUNGE AND RELISHED OUR COMMUNAL BLISS.

JIM AND I HAD SOME DAYS ALONE IN OUR SEA HOUSE. EACH TRIP TO THE LOCAL MARKET WAS AN ADVENTURE, SELECTING TOGETHER THE BEST LOCAL FARE WITH HEIGHTENED APPRECIATION FOR THE SMELLS AND TEXTURES OF SUMMER PRODUCE. EACH LUNCH OVER-LOOKING OUR SPECTACULAR VIEW OF THE MEDITERRANEAN WAS ENJOYED WITH NEW INTENSITY. OUR WALKS INTO THE TINY TOWN OF ALCÚDIA FOR A TRIP TO THE INTERNET CAFÉ AND FRESH BREAD BECAME THE MORNING ROUTINE. THE PAST CANCER-YEAR TURNED THIS ONE INTO A TIME TO LUXURIATE IN THE PULSE OF EACH DAY, EACH MEAL, EACH SUNRISE, AND EACH SUNSET. WE WERE ALIVE AND HEALTHY IN THIS SPECIAL PLACE.

AND THEN A FEW FRIENDS JOINED US FROM NASHVILLE AND PARIS, AND WE SPENT A WEEK LAUGHING AND COOKING AND PARTYING AND EXCURSIONING AND GOING OUT AGAIN ON KEVIN'S BOAT AND DIVING AGAIN AND AGAIN INTO BLUE SEA AND FEELING THE JOY AND FREEDOM OF SLICKED BACK, SALTY, WET HAIR, BEFORE THE LUNCHES ON BOARD WITH CHEESE AND WINE AND BIG, FAT, VINE-RIPE TOMATOES THAT MELT IN YOUR MOUTH. AH, THE MEDITERRANEAN DIET, EXPERIENCED WHILE FLOATING ON HER SEA.

AND THEN ON AUGUST 17, I WAS IN THE KITCHEN, PREPARING DINNER, PROBABLY CHOPPING, AND I FELT SOMETHING LUMPY UNDER MY RIGHT ARM. HALF AN ORANGE. NO, NO, NO. NO, NO, NO.

IMPRINTED ON MY BRAIN WAS DR. GREER'S REMINDER, "IT WILL COME BACK." "WHEN?" "EIGHTEEN MONTHS TO THREE YEARS." I

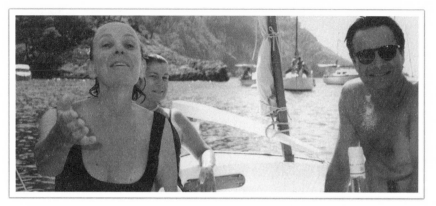

Barbara, Siggy, and Kevin on the old fishing boat.

COUNTED ON MY FINGERS. TEN MONTHS FROM THE LAST CHEMO IN OCTOBER. WAS I SUPPOSED TO START WITH THE DAY OF DIAGNOSIS, IN WHICH CASE I COULD ADD SIX MONTHS? I DIDN'T THINK SO. THIS WAS NOT GOOD NEWS.

I DIDN'T SAY ANYTHING. I GOT THROUGH DINNER. I SLEPT BADLY.

THE NEXT DAY I TOLD JIM AND WE CALLED ROY, WHO ANSWERED HIS CELL PHONE IMMEDIATELY. THANK GOD FOR THE GADGETS OF THE TWENTY-FIRST CENTURY. HIS SOOTHING VOICE AND WISE WORDS HELPED COAT MY BRAIN. HE DIDN'T THINK I WOULD NEED TO COME HOME EARLY, BUT HE WOULD CALL DR. GREER TO CONFIRM THIS DECISION AND CALL BACK.

IN THE MORNING I TOLD DANA, ONE OF OUR VISITORS FROM NASHVILLE, AND WE HUGGED AND CRIED. THE MAGIC OF THIS PLACE ACTED AS A BALM TO BUFFER AS BEST IT COULD THIS SHOCKING INVASION. THE NEXT MORNING, IN BED, I DISCOVERED ANOTHER LUMP, A WALNUT, IN MY RIGHT GROIN. GO AWAY, LEAVE ME ALONE. THE LUMPS WOULDN'T LISTEN.

I DECIDED TO PLUNGE MYSELF INTO THE LAST FOURTEEN SPANISH DAYS AND PUT FEAR AND ANXIETY ON HOLD. PICKLED WITH A FAIR AMOUNT OF WINE AND LOTS OF SALTY POTATO CHIPS, I SAW MY FRIENDS OFF, SAW JIM OFF, AND SPENT THE LAST WEEK WITH SISTER-IN-LAW, BARBARA, AND BROTHER, KEVIN, DINED AND BOATED WITH LOCAL FRIENDS, AND ON AUGUST 31, FLEW HOME.

ON THE DELTA FLIGHT FROM BARCELONA TO ATLANTA, I REGROUPED. THE LUMP WASN'T AS BIG AS BEFORE, AND IT DIDN'T HURT AS BEFORE, AND I WAS SURE IT WAS A LESSER RETURN OF THE EVIL B-CELL LYMPHOMA.

I was back home right before Labor Day. We planned to spend the holiday weekend on Monteagle Mountain, but I didn't have the strength. We cocooned at home, waiting for the Monday visit with Dr. Greer. He concurred that the disease had returned. The last hope of a large mosquito bite vanished from my brain. He scheduled a week of CAT and PET scans, and while I was in his office, brought in the pathologists for a nasty group of (where is the laughing gas when you need it?) FNA—fine-needle aspirations—the medical lingo for needle biopsies, four, probing little suckers. Bring it on. I can take it.

On Friday I got the call from Dr. Greer. The Richter's had returned. The Richter's that we had annihilated with the CHOP+R chemo last spring and fall, the procedure when I was told I was the poster child, the star of how it should be endured, where I had been given a squeaky-clean recovery profile, had returned.

This is the moment when the word "shit" is totally appropriate. Repeat three times, maybe six. In Mallorca, I kept wondering, "How do I feel about this?" Back in Nashville, I tried to write in my journal and feel the moment. But I was kind of numb. I tried to pray and felt suspended, surreal, not quite there. You think you have your life figured out, have gathered a few answers, gleaned a little wisdom and then . . . zappo, you are broadsided and back on page one.

Another visit with Dr. Greer is scheduled for the following Monday. When he opens the door to the examination room I say, "I am going to call you John on this round." I get the lowered head and shy smile, which I love. He talks about doing a new set of chemo drugs, and there are so many choices. The lead star, he thinks, will be fludarabine and the finale will be another round of Rituxan, but he doesn't commit. He will make calls to colleagues. He will discuss my unusual profile. About 5 percent of patients with CLL, chronic lympho-cytic leukemia, transform to the larger Richter's cancer at the end of a long illness, by which time they are very sick. I transformed at the beginning of my illness and I feel fine.

JIM IS THINKING ABOUT READING EVERYTHING ON THE INTERNET ABOUT EVERY CANCER DRUG AND WOULD LIKE ME TO CONSULT WITH VARIOUS OTHER MEDICAL CENTERS AROUND THE COUNTRY. I FEEL HIS MIND CHURNING, BUT THIS IS MY CALL. I AM STAYING RIGHT HERE AND LETTING JOHN AND THE OTHER JOHN (SERGENT) DO THAT RESEARCH FOR ME. THE SCIENTIFIC COMPLEXITIES OF BLOOD CANCERS ELUDE ME.

I HAVE DECIDED MY FOCUS WILL BE ON NUTRITION, BALANCE, AND GETTING MY LIFE IN A STATE OF CALM AND ORDER. AND I ALSO PLAN TO RESEARCH ALTERNATIVE, HOMEOPATHIC ROADS TO CURES. NO, I DON'T WANT TO DRIVE DR. GREER TO DRINK BUT I SENSE I WILL BE IN THIS FOR THE LONG HAUL. THE DOCTORS CAN FIGURE OUT THE DRUGS AND TREATMENT. I WILL FIGURE OUT THE BEST DIET AND EXERCISE PLAN AND INVESTIGATE AVENUES OF ALTERNATIVE HEALING.

I KNOW I HAVE THE CIRCLE OF FRIENDS DOWN PAT, THE CONTACT LIST AND AWESOME RESPONSES THAT KEEP ME GOING DOWN PAT, THE SPIRITUAL CIRCLE ON THE UPSWING. BUT, WHAT ABOUT THE REST OF MY LIFE? I MAKE CALLS TO THE NEW BOARD THAT I WAS GOING TO START—SORRY, NO; THE OLD BOARD WHERE I HAD TAKEN ON A PROJECT—SORRY, NO.

I WILL WORK WITH THE LADIES OF MAGDALENE ON JOURNAL THERAPY, AND WITH BECCA ON HER BOOK FOR OTHER CITIES THAT WANT TO TRY TO EMULATE HER INSPIRATIONAL PROGRAM, AND I WILL WRITE TO YOU AND IN MY JOURNAL TO TRY TO WRAP AROUND THE EMOTIONAL ROLLER COASTER OF CANCER, ROUND TWO.

AT HOME, I READ THE SUMMARIES OF A STUDY OF THE SUCCESS OF FLUDARABINE CHEMO ON A GROUP OF PATIENTS WITH A FIVE-YEAR REMISSION. FIVE YEARS? FIVE YEARS? I **DO NOT** THINK SO. THEY OBVIOUSLY DON'T KNOW WITH WHOM THEY ARE DEALING.

WHENEVER I CAN, I PLAN TO WALK TWO TIMES PER DAY. I AM SURE CAROLE WILL BE ALL OVER THIS WITH AN EFFICIENT SCHEDULE.

CIRCLE THE WAGONS. YOU REALLY HAVE TO BE NICE TO ME, AGAIN, FOR THE FORESEEABLE FUTURE. I AM GOING TO PONTE VEDRA FOR THE WEEK OF SEPTEMBER 18 TO GET STARTED ON BALANCE AND NUTRITION AND EXERCISE. SPA VISITS WILL BE INVOLVED.

CHEMO IS SCHEDULED FOR THE LAST WEEK IN SEPTEMBER. AND THE BEST, THE VERY BEST NEWS. MY DOCTOR "JOHN" TELLS ME THAT WITH THIS REGIMEN, I WILL NOT LOSE MY HAIR. HOW WILL I BE ABLE TO HANDLE THIS WITH NO BAD-HAIR JOKES?

LOTS OF PRAYERS ARE WELCOME AND REQUIRED. IF YOU WANT TO
GET MORE (AS EM SAYS) "DETS," YOU WILL HAVE TO SCHEDULE A WALK.

HUGS, SIGOURNEY

My editor, Beth, responds immediately with sympathy
and insight:

DEAR SIGOURNEY,

I HAD JUST SAT DOWN AT MY COMPUTER TO WRITE TO YOU. I
HEARD YOU HAD SOME NEWS VIA THE YW BOARD MEETING.

I KNOW YOU DID NOT CHOOSE TO WRITE THIS PARTICULAR
CHAPTER. BUT I THINK IT WILL GIVE YOUR BOOK A PROFOUND
IMPACT IT WOULD NOT HAVE OTHERWISE. TO BEAT IT ONCE IS A
GREAT STORY; TO TAKE THE LESSONS YOU LEARNED THE FIRST TIME
AND CONQUER ROUND TWO WILL MAKE IT EVEN STRONGER.

I AM WITH YOU ALL THE WAY.

LOVE, BETH

After sending my message into cyberspace, I go out to my garden.
The air is still summery, reasonably warm and humid in the beginning
of September, but a few brown leaves are scattered across the middle
of the green, mowed lawn. It doesn't feel like fall but the season is
creeping in, hidden behind the lush, green leaves. I hear the cat
meowing and turn to watch her walk towards me, in the grass. When
my granddaughter visits a little later in the day, she makes a beeline for
the cat, "Mimi, Mimi, where's Mimi?" The cat is nervous around little
people. I say, "Be gentle with Mimi." We reach down and stroke Mimi's
fur together. Baker has finally found a name for the cat that will stick.

When I began my first chemo, spring was coming. The garden
was opening, comforting. Now the months of chemo will be marked
by diminishing green. I walk around the crescent curve of the low
retaining wall off our bedroom thinking about another chemo and
fall. A surprising amount of flowers are still in bloom and the roses
are perking up as the temperature begins to cool down. How will it
feel to watch the flowers return to the earth rather than bloom and

grow as I tackle another six months of chemo? Fall is a harvest. The black walnut tree leaning over the roof will begin to drop big, fat nuts that roll down the slanted tile roof of our house in the middle of the night. Maybe I will have time to pickle some of the crab apples from the trees on the front lawn. But nothing will distract me from the return of the dreaded Richter's syndrome, the nasty one that is supposed to be gone forever. Dr. Greer has already planted the seed about the possible next step to stem-cell transplant. He suggests I concentrate on the chemo now and think about transplants later. Yeah, right. For sure, more challenges await.

I go and sit on the side porch and open to page 28 of my new book, *Absolute Beginner's Guide to Alternative Medicine,* by Karen L. Fontaine. Both Dr. Johns are uncomfortable with unscientific cures, yet my nurse practitioner buddy, Ellen, is a strong supporter of homeopathic practices and cancer-friendly diets. Ellen and I will conspire together. I am already in touch with a trainer and dietician at Vanderbilt. The reality check from round two means fitness and diet will become important regimens for the rest of my time.

I should be terrified, trembling. Yet the truth is there has never been a moment when I wasn't sure I would survive.

Maybe it's just the default mind-set—a universal strain—I will live. Our minds are set on forward until we are so close to the final door we can reach out, touch it, and know the other side, death, is the only option left. Lots of life has to be used up before stepping towards the last threshold. And I suspect the majority of the players are dragged through struggling to resist.

I plan to take my time, allowing significant climbs and curves and practice rounds and explorations into every nook and cranny before I am ready to say, "It is time," and then, I hope, I can enter the final door with just a whisper of grace.

Epilogue

My book ends with a second lump and the first thing people want to know is how I am. I didn't mean to set up a cliff-hanger.

The answer is, I am fine. I have been in remission for 14 months. The second diagnosis was another round of the dreaded Richter's Syndrome, another operation to put the port back in (which I was never going to need again as I had sailed through the first chemo round leaving no trace of disease) and another round of six months of chemo, every three weeks, and another six months of being sick and life on hold. But, wait a minute, I didn't really put life on hold. If you have read my book, you have figured out I'm not capable of putting life on hold and am convinced living life as normally as possible helps the healing process. So, in January Jim and I went to New Zealand to visit our son, Daniel and his new bride, Anne, where they spent the first year of marriage with Daniel practicing his first year of emergency medicine in the charming town of Rotarua. Then, we went to Sydney, staying at the Park Hyatt, almost under the Harbour Bridge with panoramic views of the opera house. We watched the Australian Open Tennis Tournament and walked for miles each day. In March I went skiing and made some pretty good runs, keeping up with my other children, Jamie and Lisa and Matthew and Jessie. Well, they had to wait for me from time to time at the base of a steep slope and I didn't last too long, but I was there with the sticks pointed down the hill.

My team of email friends increases as I tour the country with *Patient Siggy* and my heart sings with added rhythm as I add each name. I use the trip as a perfect excuse to reconnect with many old friends from high school and college. As I write these words, my contact list just hit 600.

I find that I'm a ham. I love talking in front of an audience and I try to make each book appearance slightly different. Sometimes I dwell on the spiritual side of my journey, other times on the emergence of my writing, other times on the power behind my circle of friends. I focused on Grandpa Jim when I spoke at his retirement community. I was asked to fill the spot for the Spanish program at a local woman's club so I put together a PowerPoint slide show and talked about growing up on the island of Mallorca. I've been to California and New York and Connecticut and Washington and even London. Sometimes my audience is 150 and sometimes it is 8. The audience of 8 asked the best questions.

I see a specialist in my disease at Sloan Kettering in New York every four months and I see Dr. Greer at Vanderbilt in between. They didn't take the port out this time, so I have the half-dollar lump in my chest, just below my right collarbone as a reminder that I need to stay in the moment each day. Don't worry about a thing. I plan to live to 80. Oh, and I'm half way through the next book.

Got to go. Here comes another email from a new fan from London asking to be put on the list. That's 601.

Reactions and Reflections

Comments from my readers suggest themes for discussion and reflection. Comments followed by stars were emails.

Living Each Day "This book is not about cancer. It is about how to live! Your journey has lighted the way for the rest of us." Cathy

Heal Others and Heal Yourself "As a nurse I have known I couldn't ever really 'fix' anybody, but I have tried to stand 'in the ditch' with my patients. I have tried to be a 'helper-guide' and not look away even if a patient's journey through diagnosis and treatment didn't take them back to health as we hoped it would. Cancer and the unknown are some of the things we humans fear the most. All I've ever wanted as a nurse was to have a pair of hands that can be useful. As you discovered long ago when you were fighting depression, the way to real happiness is through service to others." Ellen

The Power of Prayer "When my husband died I could not pray. I was crushed, bewildered and angry, angry. Sometime later when I was alone the silence you describe so beautifully brought me peace. I could connect with God again and tearfully ask His help. Your book is such a blessing, to those who have had bad things happen to them. Drifting from pain to the beauty of your garden, love of friends and touches of humor are a lesson in courage. I prayed for you when I first learned of your illness. I pray for you now. God will listen." Dora

Appearances The first question a person may ask when diagnosed with cancer is, Will I lose my hair? "When you lose your hair, accept the loss of vanity; you're just getting closer to the real you—the Sigourney inside—the part that really matters to everyone who knows and cares for you." Jane

Suffering Understood "I have just read *Patient Siggy* in its entirety in less than 24 hours, an all-time first for me. I feel compelled to let you know how much I relate to what you had to say without my being a cancer victim. I feel certain that most other non-cancer readers around my age will feel the same. Your book, for me, is all about coping with the trials and tribulations of living, particularly when one is 'slam-dunked' by a major crisis." Kay. She encloses another Henri Nouwen quotation: "When we honestly ask ourselves which persons in our lives mean the most to us, we often find it is those who instead of cures, have chosen rather to SHARE OUR PAIN AND TOUCH OUR WOUNDS WITH A GENTLE AND TENDER HAND."

Intimacy "The power of your story is that you open a door and bring us into your life with frankness and honesty. We feel privileged that we know you so well and thus . . . know ourselves." Guna.

Courage and Vulnerability "I took your book to bed. My husband asked how long I was going to read. I replied, 'As long as I can.' At page 87 I folded, but your story woke me long before dawn ricocheting around in my head and I read on. Your honesty and bravery and vulnerability touch me. The problem for you now is that you have let so many into your heart, your body and your soul that when we greet you, we know you so much more than you know us. I have to think about how that feels." Judy

Priorities "The best is the reflection of where you go now. It is thought-provoking, not just for the patients who have cancer or any disease, or tribulation, but for all of us who need to be more reflective about where our lives are heading." Carole★★

Community Healing "I have just finished reading your book and it has been a gift for me. I came to your book signing in London and am a friend of our host, Missy. Please add me to your circle of friends. I love the idea of staying connected as your journey continues. Stay well." Jacquie

Finding a Voice for Illness "My best friend was just diagnosed with cancer. I didn't know how to talk to her but after reading your book I do." Faith

Being Heard "Opening your heart to others allows them to be opened back. We all hunger for this connectedness. Henri Nouwen reminds us, 'As a human being, our greatest desire is to be known.'" Janet

Blessings "Finding your beautiful email last night I was so moved. As you feel blessed by others' care and attention, you need to know what a blessing your writing is to those of us receiving it. Your tender, honest words remind us all, of the daily gifts we take for granted. They have urged me to stop and notice the love and beauty all around me in ways I don't, due to business. That business, I must realize, is my choice. Therefore, I can—and must—choose more wisely. Thank you for the lesson." Beth★★

Coming Home "You have found your voice. Your details are as well chosen as the objects in your living room." Alice

Women Power "I have come up with the answer to an eternal, heretofore unanswered question that has haunted humanity forever: Why do women live longer than men? It's simple: You girls stick together. When one of you is down, the herd comes to the rescue." Randy

The Gift of Sharing "Your book is addicting. I am going to be late because I couldn't resist picking it up this morning and then I couldn't stop reading. It's like talking to you at your most eloquent, with all of your descriptions filling in the edges and putting us inside you. I can't wait to finish it but don't want it to end. You have given us all a wonderful, special gift." Varina

The Gift of Cancer "There are so many sweet blessings that come about with having cancer. Truthfully, I gained much more than I had to suffer, and life, friends, and my family all are part of what I treasure most now. God is good to us. He allows our suffering but offers peace and blessings that flow through the love and care of others. You will be changed forever." Another Cathy★★

The Power of Community "I believe that in a volunteer community of friends praying for one another, the greatest wealth of life is experienced." Becca

About the Author

*S*igourney Woods Cheek earned a bachelor's degree in art history from Manhattanville College and studied on the graduate level at Vanderbilt University. Active for many years in the Nashville fine arts community, she co-founded the Antiques and Garden Show as a fundraiser for Cheekwood and the Exchange Club of Nashville. She has chaired the Iroquois Steeplechase, the Swan Ball, and the board of directors of Cheekwood Botanical Gardens and Fine Arts Center. Cheek has also served on the boards of the Junior League of Nashville, Leadership Nashville Alumni, Nashville Institute for the Arts, the Garden Club of Nashville, and Belle Meade Metro Planning Commission. She currently serves on the boards of the YWCA, Cheekwood Botanical Gardens, the Antique and Garden Show of Nashville, the Vestry of Christ Church Cathedral, and Magdalene House, for which she also conducts writing workshops for women in recovery. She and her husband, James H. Cheek III, reside in Nashville; they have three sons and two grandchildren.

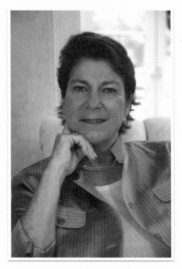

Photo: Kimberly Manz